GW00859248

# I Want Sex, *He Wants Fries*

## *5-Step Plan to Beat Low Testosterone & Get Your Sex Life Back on Track*

## Rebecca Watson

DISCLAIMER: This book is not intended to be a substitute for medical advice; in fact, one of its primary purposes is to help you find the medical professionals who can help you.

In this book I offer information based on my work with individuals and couples struggling in low testosterone marriages; however, not everything works for everybody.

Before implementing any of the medical suggestions in this book, please check with your doctor to make sure they're right for you.

Readers hold the author harmless for negative outcomes based on following the suggestions in this book. Each marriage is different and not every strategy in this book will be right for you and your marriage.

Copyright © 2015 Rebecca Watson

All rights reserved.

ISBN:1514125242

ISBN-13:9781514125243

To all those low T couples struggling to hold
their marriages together

Hang in there, there's light at the end of the
tunnel.

# TABLE OF CONTENTS

# Foreword

For the good wife, who enjoys sex, having a low T husband is its own private hell.

There's no good way to talk to your friends about your husband's sexual problems. It just invites a barrage of the most personal questions, for which you really have no answers. Your friends and family aren't able to help, he doesn't want to talk about it, and the resources out there for the wives of low T husbands are nearly non-existent. In addition, low T tends to sneak into a good relationship unannounced, veiled in a fog of small excuses, white lies and confusion. Half the reason you can't talk about it is you're just wondering if the real problem is you.

When I first met Rebecca, her husband had already started testosterone therapy, but the six years of confusion and repeated sexual rejection had torn her apart. There was treatment for him, but not treatment for her.

Which is why in desperation she contacted me via my blog, and spilled the entire story. The pain. The doctors. The rejection. The awkward failures. The gnawing temptation to just walk away from the pride-swallowing siege and start over.

I read her email over and replied. I finished my email with...

"I think you've done the right thing in holding up your end of the marriage and giving him a fair warning and getting him into treatment. For what it's worth, I'm proud of you."

For me it was a throwaway line. I'm proud of you. It sounded good, so I said it. For her, it was a lifeline in the midst of feeling thrown away.

"I actually cried when I read that. I didn't realize how much I needed to hear it. It has been so *hard* to keep going in this marriage, and my husband hasn't been able to give me a lot of support because he's struggling himself to come to terms with the whole situation."

I would love to say that my email magically fixed everything, but it did mark a turning point. In the early days, there were still some remarkably emotional and dramatic moments, but she also showed so much heart I always felt like she was going to make it through.

Then as her own pain started to subside, her compassion for others started to shine. There was no requirement that she help anyone else but herself, but she stayed in the game anyway. She became my first moderator on my forum. Then a year later, she joined me as a life coach and now specializes in low T couples.

Why you need this book:

(1)    Rebecca's knowledge of testosterone is encyclopedic, but she always keeps it simple to understand, and easy to put the next step into action. You aren't going to get lost in jargon.

(2)    She knows what it's like being in your situation. She's cried alone in the bathroom wearing lingerie too. This isn't an academic exercise for her, she genuinely cares that you get the help you need.

(3)    She understands that it all doesn't just end with riding off into the sunset after your husband gets on medication. There's so much that comes after that to relearn your relationship that your doctors simply won't know about, even assuming there was time in a 15-minute appointment to cover it.

(4)    There's nothing else out there for wives. To be sure, there are some dry medical tomes about testosterone, but nothing else really acknowledges the wife's perspective and struggle. She's written the book she could have used all those years ago.

So think of Rebecca as your big sister who went through it all before you. She can't magically fix low T, but she will probably save you a couple of years of trial and error, maybe save your marriage, and definitely save your sanity.

**Athol Kay**
**Professional Married Guy**

# Acknowledgments

First and foremost, I want to thank Athol Kay for his unfailing mentorship and support as I wrote this book. He encouraged, edited, pushed, prodded and poked; and cracked the whip when I slacked off.

He gave of his time, his effort, and his energy. He never lost faith that I would complete this work, and for that he has my utmost gratitude. This book would not exist without him.

I also want to thank the women in my life who encouraged and supported me in the writing of this book. My mom, Shirley Watson, whose courage in starting a new career in the second half of her life inspired me to take on this challenge. She has provided love and support every step of the way. My sister, Debra Watson, and sister-in-law, Nancy Inman, who spurred me on. My lovely niece, Danielle Marrazzo, whose enthusiasm for this project buoyed my spirits. My friend, Helen Hart, who continually lifted me up in this endeavor and whose technical support was invaluable.

I am thankful for my dad, Charles Watson, whose unflinching example of honor, integrity and strength kept my feet on a straight path when they wanted to stray.

A huge thank you to Kathleen Alkema, whose edits made this book tighter, cleaner and easier to read; and to Brian Rideout and Jennifer Kay for generously sharing information and technical support.

*Acknowledgments*

My special thanks goes to the men and women I've worked with who are struggling in low T marriages. Their courage and commitment in the face of adversity is heartwarming. They have entrusted me with their stories and struggles and I have learned so much from them. My hope is that this book justifies their trust.

To my children, who gave up hot meals and clean clothes so that I could finish this book. They were willing to forego the time and attention of their mom and fill in the gaps, and for that I am grateful.

Watching their peacefully sleeping faces kept me from giving up during a dark place in my marriage. I am so much richer for having them in my life.

And finally, to my husband, Ron.

From the moment I asked him about writing this book, he has given constant encouragement and support. He's offered suggestions and feedback, and listened patiently while I've read chapters aloud. He's helped me understand the point-of-view of the guy who is sharing this struggle with his wife, and his input has been invaluable.

Moreover, he had the courage to allow me to share our very personal story with others ... not an easy thing to do.

He never lost hope for our marriage even at a time when I did. He had the perseverance and strength to prevail and for that, I am very thankful.

# Introduction

## He'd Rather Have Fries than Sex

Are you tired of lying awake at night, listening to your husband's peaceful, even breathing, hoping that this will be the night that he (finally) initiates sex? Are you longing for him to look at you again with that glint in his eyes that reminds you that he's a man and you're a woman? Do you have to hold back tears as you walk through the lingerie department, looking wistfully at all the pretty things, but knowing that your husband wouldn't bother to glance up from the TV even if you paraded in front of him stark naked?

## You Are Not Alone

If your husband is thinking french fries while you're thinking sex, you are not alone. One of the worst things about being married to a guy whose interest in sex has disappeared is that you don't have anyone to talk to about the problem and don't know where to turn for answers.

While you may feel like you're the only one in the world with this problem, I can promise you that you're not. I talk with women every day who are in the same situation and who are taking steps to reclaim the desire and intimacy in their marriage.

## Five Basic Questions

There are five basic questions a woman asks when her husband's sex drive goes away.

- *Why doesn't my husband want to have sex with me?*
- *What is wrong with him?*
- *What is wrong with **me**?*
- *Does he have someone else?*

- *Is it going to get better or am I doomed to live this way for the rest of my life?*

I wrote this book to answer those questions and save others the many years and thousands of dollars my husband and I wasted on dead-end solutions and advice from misinformed professionals. I want to help you avoid adding to the gaping emotional wounds your marriage has already suffered and speed you along the way with fewer detours.

## Taking the Fear Out of Low Testosterone

Low testosterone is one of those phrases that strikes fear into a man's heart. He feels like he's too young to have to worry about testosterone levels. But T levels can drop for all sorts of reasons and in men of all ages.

In fact, one estimate is that almost **one in four men over the age of 30 has clinically low testosterone levels**!

# A Man Doesn't Stop Wanting Sex for No Reason

If your husband's sex drive has diminished, there's a reason. It's not that he's simply getting older, it's not that it's normal for married couples to stop having sex, it's not that you two are getting 'too old for that sort of thing'.

My guess is that you're reading these words with a mixture of hope, desperation and despair. By the time a woman starts searching for the reasons behind her husband's missing sex drive, she has usually hit her breaking point. Several years ago, I hit mine.

# The Long Journey

Last night, my husband tossed me down on the bed and made mad passionate love to me. Six years ago, if you had told me I would ever write those words, I would have laughed. Or cried.

Six years ago, my marriage was in a very dark place, empty of passion and excitement. While I craved emotional connection and sexual release with my husband, he was uninterested, withdrawn and apathetic, completely oblivious to my body. I tried everything I knew to revive his interest, but nothing worked. I was faced with the dismal prospect of living like roommates for the rest of my life.

*The rest of my life.* Those words haunted me. I felt young and vibrant, and now that our baby years were behind us, I had never felt more sexual. How could I possibly survive the next thirty years with a guy who treated me like a congenial roommate?

For years, I stumbled around looking for answers, meeting dead ends and feeling sorry for myself as our marriage died ... one pathetic encounter at a time. It wasn't until the night he fell asleep during foreplay and I sobbed by the bathtub that I finally got serious about looking for a solution.

# Finding Answers

I was faced with a mystery. When I first met my husband, he was a vibrant, energetic guy with a zest for life. He couldn't wait to jump me any chance he got. What happened to take him from that to a guy who would rather watch infomercials than have sex with me? Solving this mystery took me on a long journey and ended in a surprising destination.

# Solving the Mystery

It turned out that the reason for my husband's lagging sex drive and lack of energy was a hormonal imbalance. He had the testosterone levels of an eighty-year-old man! Suddenly, his behavior started making sense.

During my search for answers, I stumbled across other women struggling in the same dark place I had been. What surprised me most was the sheer number of men and women who were dealing with this issue and the amount of pain and damage low testosterone was inflicting in their marriages. All this time, I had thought I was alone, but I was just one of many.

# The Low T Script

As my husband and I pulled ourselves out of the low T pit, I started putting my knowledge to use to help other couples avoid all the pitfalls we had encountered along the way.

As I coached couples in low T marriages, I was struck by how similar their stories were; in fact, it was like reading from a script. There were the same challenges, the same ups and downs, and the same responses.

I quickly realized that most couples had no idea how to fix the problem, and in fact, were actually acting in ways that made it worse.

This mirrored my own experiences in restoring my low T marriage. Even after my husband and I addressed the medical issues, we faced a number of challenges in putting our marriage back together and we made many blunders along the way. In fact, on the list of *Things **Not** to Do to Fix Your Low T Marriage*, I'm pretty sure we managed to check off most of the boxes.

We wasted several years and thousands of dollars on wrong turns; I'd like to help you avoid all that.

Having lived through it all and after having spent two years coaching couples in low T marriages, I can see five very predictable stages of recovery that happen with everyone. Each stage has its own challenges, but they really do read like a script. Knowing the script is 80% of the battle and will save you time, money and a lot of painful moments with each other.

# What You Can Expect in this Book

This book is not a warm and fuzzy feel-good book; it's a nitty-gritty survival manual with practical tips and information to let you quickly take action to fix the problem. You don't need more talk; you need action! This is the book I wish I would have had during the darks years in our marriage when we were flailing around, searching for answers.

**Stage One** – Solving the mystery of the missing libido

- *Common symptoms of low testosterone*
- *How do you know whether low T is really affecting his sex drive*
- *The simple test that tells you for sure whether low T is an issue*
- *How to get lab work done the quickest, easiest way possible*
- *How to get your husband on board*
- *What it means when the doctor says his levels are 'normal' (Hint: It doesn't mean what you think it means.)*
- *Health implications of low T*

**Stage Two** – How testosterone production goes wrong and what you can do about it

- *Can he **really** increase his T levels naturally*
- *What caused his low T levels*
- *How to save time and money on finding a doctor who knows what they're doing*
- *Learning the jargon you need to know to talk to the doctor*
- *Why you shouldn't rush into T therapy immediately*

**Stage Three** – Fixing the medical the quickest, easiest, safest way possible

- *How to save money on lab work and treatment plans*
- *The most convenient and effective treatment options*
- *What you need to know to keep testosterone treatment safe*
- *How long does it take to see results after T therapy*
- *What to do about erectile dysfunction*

**Stage Four** – A step-by-step blueprint to get your marriage and sex life back on track as quickly as possible

- *Why your sex life doesn't immediately bounce back after T therapy*
- *The #1 thing you are doing that reduces his interest*
- *Tools that get you back on the same team*
- *Why he stalks you like a lion does a gazelle in the morning, only to fade away by nighttime*
- *What you're doing in the bedroom that is killing your sex life*
- *The setback that you will inevitably encounter and how to keep it from derailing your progress*

**Stage Five** - High T Marriage

- *How you and your husband are not the same people you were before low T*
- *Why your husband values you more now than he did*
- *Wow, he never used to do **that** in the bedroom!*
- *Falling in love with your husband all over again*

**Throughout the Book**

- *Real stories from real people who have successfully navigated the low T waters*
- *Information and tips from top doctors and researchers in the field*
- *Glossary of medical terms you need to know to effectively communicate with the doctor*

# Let's Get Started!

You've spent enough time crying by the bathtub in your lingerie. The quicker we get started, the quicker you're going to regain the sexual energy and emotional intimacy you crave with your husband. Let's get the ball rolling and get your marriage back on track!

# For Men Only

## If Your Wife Just Handed You This Book …

… I know how you feel.

Hi, my name is Ron, and my wife's name is Rebecca; she's the author of the book you're holding.

I've been where you are. I was the guy who ignored all my symptoms and tried to pretend that everything was okay. My wife had talked to me until she was blue in the face about seeing a doctor for my low T symptoms, but I'm a stubborn guy; I didn't budge. In fact, the more she talked about it, the angrier and more stubborn I got. I wanted her to just *leave it alone.*

At my wife's urging, I finally asked my doctor about T therapy and the only thing he told me was that it would shrink my testicles. That didn't sound good. I also had it in my head that it would cause prostate cancer. (It doesn't, by the way.) I hated the idea that I had to take some type of medicine in order to be a man. It seemed like an admission of failure, and my main thought was, "Hell, no."

So there I was digging in my heels, and there she was miserable in our marriage. It wasn't until she came to me and told me that she couldn't live like this anymore that things changed. She had said those words before, but this time something was different. This time, I could tell she meant it.

That was the slap in the head it took for me to finally face the fact that I could lose my marriage if I kept ignoring the problem.

I wasn't happy about it. To be honest, I was mad as hell. I hated feeling like she had cornered me into doing something I didn't want to do. I hated the idea of being hooked on some kind of drug forever. But … I also love my wife. I didn't want to lose her.

So I made the appointment, one thing led to another, and I started T therapy. I wish you could see for yourself the difference it's made in my life. I didn't even realize how bad I was feeling until I started feeling better. It was the difference in going from black and white to color.

I lost weight, built muscle, gained energy and actually wanted to jump my beautiful wife again. It's like I turned the clock back twenty years! Nowadays, I take a mixed martial arts class, work out in the gym at my office, and have my life back. I finally feel like a *man* again! My only regret about T therapy is that I waited so long to start it.

You may be as stubborn as I am, in which case nothing I say will make a difference, but my advice to you is to read this book with an open mind. Separate out the truth about testosterone from the myths you've heard.

If your T levels are low, you're living half a life. You're tired and unmotivated. Your memory has turned to crap and you have a hard time focusing. Your arms are getting smaller and your gut is getting bigger.

And if your wife has searched out this book, your marriage is going downhill fast. I know the idea of taking a med in order 'to be a man' makes you feel old and weak, but the truth is that you're already feeling old and weak because of your T levels.

If your wife is still pestering you about this, it means she loves you and hasn't given up on the marriage. Take the ball and run with it. Get her to find you a good doctor and go see what he says. You have nothing to lose and everything to gain.

Best of luck, Ron

# Stage One

# The Mystery of the Missing Libido

*The Early Years*

Sunlight streamed through the window, and my husband's hand slipped lower, knowing exactly what to do to push me to the edge as I squirmed in my seat, the seatbelt getting in the way,

"Stop it," I laughed. "You need to concentrate on the road. You're going to get us both killed."

"I'm better driving with one hand than you are with two," he responded, his hand never hesitating. I shifted in the seat to give him better access, my eyes drifting shut.

He grinned, loving the way he could push me into losing my inhibitions, and then caught my hand in his, pulling it toward him. Part of what I loved about him was that wild streak that appealed to my love of adventure.

With only ten minutes left to go in our trip, I pushed his hand away and started to put myself back together, not wanting to arrive at his family's flushed and embarrassed.

Upstairs, as I set out our toiletries in the bathroom, my husband pushed the door open to join me. He closed the door behind him and pulled me to him, kissing and stroking.

"Stop it! Do **not** get me going again when you know it's going to be hours before we get to bed."

He laughed and started undoing snaps and zippers.

"What are you doing? Your family is right downstairs!" I said as I frantically tried to remember the layout of the house, calculating what room we were above and who might be below us to hear.

"Shhhh..... I don't care about my family or what they're doing. What I care about is my wife. Just relax and let go," he murmured as he spread a towel on the cold bathroom tile.

### The Dark Years

My husband's hand stroked gently over my bare shoulders and down my side. I tried to relax into the moment, but things had been bad between us for so long. So many fights and tears over our lack of sex life. He had suggested a sexual massage as a peace offering, and I wanted so much to enjoy it; I was starved for sex and physical touch, but knowing he was doing it *for me* as a sort of consolation prize killed much of the enjoyment.

I sighed and let my eyes close as his hands evoked a response from my body, if not my mind, feeling pleasure rising as his hands moved lower. He moved slower and slower and I shifted restlessly, wanting more. His hand slowed to a stop and I opened my eyes, trying to see through the darkness to determine what he was doing. His snore jerked him awake and he started.

"Did you fall **asleep**?" my voice rose incredulously.

"No!" he said and then stopped, knowing there was no response he could give that would make the moment any better. His hands started rubbing again as he tried to ignore the situation and pretend it hadn't happened, but I pushed him away.

I went into the bathroom, closing the door behind me and knelt by the bathtub, sobbing.

# Chapter 1

# Your Sex Life Is AWOL
## *The Fog*

I knew my marriage was in trouble the night I dressed up in his favorite French maid outfit and he started having passionate thoughts  about ... *french fries*. And when I bent over the bed, he gazed at my buns and thought longingly of two all-beef patties with special sauce. It got so bad that his idea of a hot date was adding tabasco sauce to his chili dog.

Nearly any kind of TV was enough of a distraction from sex for him too. A good rerun of *Friends* would do it ... or even a bad one. I remember one night he told me to take a bath, he would be right in ... *wink wink, nudge nudge* ... 45 minutes later, shriveled and shivering, I squelched soggily into the living room to find him engrossed in an infomercial for vacuum cleaners. Something about that self-adjusting cleaner head with the powerful motorized brush had him completely enthralled. "Oh, sorry," he said. "I lost track of time."

That was ... strange. I felt a tiny chill run down my spine. Just that slightest hint that something was off although I wasn't sure what. What I didn't know at the time was that this night would mark the beginning of a long and difficult chapter in our marriage.

It was like one day I just looked up and realized that my husband's sex drive was AWOL and without realizing it, we had turned into roommates. While he was still warm and loving with me, he simply didn't seem physically attracted to me in the same way he used to be. Night after night, he was content to snuggle with me on the sofa instead of taking me in the bedroom and tossing me down on the bed. I had never signed up to be roommates!

Along with his missing libido, some other things had disappeared ... his energy, his motivation, and his sense of fun. He spent a lot more time falling asleep in front of the TV than he used to. While *he* chalked it up to a stressful job and getting older, *I* knew there had to be more to it than that. He was too young to feel so old!

## Looking for Clues

If this is going on in your marriage, you are probably just as confused as I was. It's kind of like you have your own personal version of *Invasion of the Body Snatchers* going on and you're wondering who took your real husband and left behind this hollow shell of a man. He's definitely not the same guy you married. You want to say ... *whoever stole my husband, would you please give him back*?

You can see that he's struggling, but you don't know how to help. He drudges through his day, just trying to put one foot in front of the other. You're torn between compassion and the desire to *wring his neck*! Because my gosh, the way he shuffles and sighs and constantly falls asleep in front of the TV is driving you nuts! You're tempted to check his pulse once in a while just to make sure he's still alive.

And sex? Well, his sex drive seems to be missing in action. It shows up once in a while if the planets align in just the right way but that guy who couldn't wait to pounce on you is nowhere to be seen. Where did he go? It's a mystery.

Maybe you're wondering if he's found someone else. But then again, where would he find the energy? You've wondered if he's gay, but that doesn't fit either. Alternative life styles take a lot of effort, and he isn't motivated to do much of *anything* lately. Or maybe he simply doesn't find you attractive anymore. There have been a few times where he seemed up for sex, but his equipment ...wasn't. *Ouch.* That killed the deal ... for both of you. You lie in bed at night listening to him breathe, wanting to shake the answers out of him.

## Missing Libido

So you've got this mystery on your hands that you can't figure out, with you and your husband reluctantly playing the lead roles. You've talked to your husband about what's going on, but he doesn't have any answers; heck, he doesn't even seem to recognize that there's a problem. "I'm just tired, honey."

He says it's *normal* for couples to stop having sex after they've been married as long as you have. *You* see it as this huge red flag that something is wrong; *he* sees it as a normal passage of life. You wonder which of you is right. You've started questioning whether there's something wrong with *you* that you miss sex so much. He acts like he's a dinosaur while you feel young and vibrant.

## Marriage Is a Sexual Union

But here's the deal ... at its heart, marriage is a sexual union.

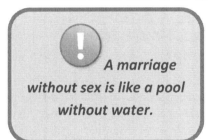

*A marriage without sex is like a pool without water.*

Without sex, you have a roommate, not a marriage. A marriage without sex is like a pool without water ... empty and disappointing. If you're not getting sex in your marriage, then in a very real sense you are being cheated out of what you signed up for. There was a time when your husband would have been first in line to agree with that statement. What happened to that guy?

## No One to Talk To

By this point, you probably feel like you have nowhere to turn. You need his help to solve the mystery, but he simply doesn't want to talk about it. If your husband is like most men struggling with low desire, he may have reached the point where he gets defensive and irritated any time you bring it up. He tells you that if you would just stop nagging him so much, maybe he would want it more. Oh *right*, like that's worked so well for you! It's just his way of avoiding a topic that makes him feel inadequate. The problem is that if you *do* talk about not having sex, he doesn't want sex ... and if you *don't* talk about not having sex, he doesn't want sex. Hmmm ... where's the winning combination here?

Okay, you can't talk to your husband about what's going on, but you need to talk to *someone*! Your best friend? Um, *no*. If she talks about sex at all, it's to complain that her husband is constantly wanting it, no matter how tired she is. Your mom? Your sister? Could there be a more embarrassing conversation than to admit that your husband has lost interest in you? Nope, there's no help there.

Maybe you've thought about making a doctor appointment for him, but what kind of doctor should it be and what would you say? "My husband is tired all the time and would rather have Cheetos than have me." You flinch when you think about having that particular conversation. You're not sure how you would get your husband to go to the doctor anyway, when he doesn't even admit there's a problem. You just don't know what else to do.

You probably feel fairly discouraged right about now, but hang on because there's help to be had. If your guy would rather bury his face in a box of glazed donuts than between your breasts, then keep reading; this book is for you.

## Identifying the Culprit

Here's the thing you need to understand. A man's libido doesn't disappear for no reason. I'll pause to let that sink in. *A man's libido doesn't disappear for no reason.* I know, I just used a double negative. Meaning that there *is* a reason for the change in his sex drive. Even though you don't yet know what it is, there is an underlying cause for his missing libido. While you

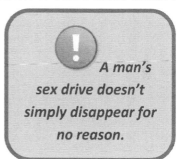

*A man's sex drive doesn't simply disappear for no reason.*

may feel powerless at this point to solve the mystery, you actually have a vital role to play in finding the answers and fixing the problem.

So what could it be? What's causing his sex drive and energy to tank? You've taken stock of the situation and ruled out the more obvious culprits; he's not having an affair, he's not gay, he doesn't seem to be depressed, and he's not addicted to porn. What's left?

Well, it's possible that what you're dealing with is a hormonal problem called low testosterone. That sounds all sinister and scary, but low testosterone is actually fairly simple to treat. Of all the things that can affect energy and sex drive, low testosterone is by far one of the

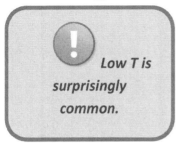

Low T is surprisingly common.

most common, and compared to an affair, et al., it's also the easiest to deal with.

In fact, low T is surprisingly common; in one study of 1475 men with a mean age of 47.3, 24% of the men had low testosterone levels (defined as less than 300ng/dL). Testosterone levels decline with age, so low T becomes increasingly more prevalent as men get older. While not all men with low T levels experience symptoms, for a sizable number of them low T is a libido killer. When those testosterone levels go down, sex drive quickly follows.

## You're Not Crazy

When you're in the dark years of low testosterone, it's easy to forget what things used to be like for you and your husband. You start questioning whether your memories of how things used to be are even accurate. You start feeling like things have always been this way and always will be ... especially if your husband is living in denial, and tells you that it's normal for couples to stop being intimate after they've been married a while.

He'll say things like, "Honey, we're not 26 anymore. Every guy I know is tired all the time and no one I know who's been married for this many years has all that much sex." And you start thinking, "Maybe he's right. Maybe *I'm* the one who's being unreasonable. But if he's right, then why am I so miserable?"

Memories of encounters we had from earlier in our marriage are what sustained me during the darkest times when my husband was deep in the low T fog. When I was ready to give up on my marriage, my memories gave me hope. I knew that somewhere behind that tired, run-down, passionless façade, was the bold, sexy, sensual man I had married. I knew that things could be different for us. At times, that hope was the only thing that kept me going.

What I want you to do is to pull up a memory from when your husband was sexy, confident and vibrant, and I want you to hold on to that when things get bad. That guy is still there. He's hiding under all the low T layers, but he's there. The trick is finding him again.

## Round-Up of Symptoms

Okay, let's put it all together. While your frustrated nights are probably what drove you here, they're not the only problem. Guys with low testosterone levels usually have a boatload of other things going on; low energy, lack of motivation, trouble concentrating and remembering, weight gain and muscle loss, and problems with erections. They simply seem to lose their zest for life. I've included a Low T quiz at the end of the chapter so you can check to see whether your husband has any low T symptoms.

Adam experienced low T as a flatlining:

*"I just feel gray all the time. I don't get excited about things the way I used to. I go to work, I come home, I watch TV, and I go to bed. Every day is the same. Nothing seems worth a lot of effort anymore."*

*--Adam, Investment Analyst, 39*

For Jeff, it was the fatigue that got to him:

*"When I was low T, my energy was low; I woke up late, ran out of energy early and couldn't focus easily. I was able to get through my day and get my work done, but it took all I had. There was no extra capacity for thinking ahead or making plans. The bedroom was actually the last place I saw symptoms. The mental fog and afternoon fatigue came much earlier.*

*Jeff, 43, Sales Manager*

## Unique Man - Unique Symptoms

It's important to note that not every man reacts to low T in the same way. I've worked with guys whose libido stayed high even while energy and concentration took a nosedive. Some guys who start out with a high sex drive may go from wanting sex seven times a week to only wanting it three times a week. Or a guy may go from initiating frequently to waiting until his wife initiates. Another guy may not only not initiate, he may actually turn his wife down when she initiates.

> **Low T creeps up gradually and subtly, unnoticed at first by either partner.**

Some guys notice an inability to concentrate or a feeling of depression first, while others notice a lack of energy. I've worked with guys at 200ng/dL who could barely get out of bed; I've also worked with guys who were quite functional at the same level. It simply depends on the individual man.

Mike had no idea how low testosterone had impacted him until *after* he started T therapy.

*"I didn't realize how much low T was affecting me until I increased my levels. Now I can look back and see how many areas of my life were impacted, but if you had asked me at the time, I would have told you that I felt fine. I feel alive again."*

—*Mike, 53, Compensation Manager*

Low testosterone affects multiple areas of a man's life. Take a look at the questions below and see if they ring a bell.

---

## The Low T Quiz

☐ *Have you noticed that his sex drive isn't as strong as it used to be?*

☐ *Does your husband seem tired a lot, even though he's getting plenty of sleep?*

☐ *Is he less fun; the things he used to love to do are too much bother now? Is he less social than he used to be?*

☐ *Is he finding it more difficult to concentrate and forgets things more often than he used to?*

☐ *Is he grumpy, stressed, moody or irritable more often than he used to be?*

☐ *Have you noticed that his morning erections are less frequent or less firm?*

☐ *Does he lose his erection more often than he used to? Are his erections less firm?*

☐ *Is he having a tough time losing weight, with a lot of his weight primarily in his mid-section?*

☐ *Is he having a tough time gaining muscle, even though he's working out?*

---

Does a lot of this sound familiar? If your husband is dealing with some of these symptoms, the culprit may be low testosterone. So you can put away those sharp implements. It's not that he's lazy; it's not that he doesn't love you; it's not that he finds you unattractive. He doesn't have a girl … or a guy … stashed away somewhere. His hormones are simply messed up.

As one of my low T clients told me, "During the worst of my low T phase, Salma Hayek could have stood in front of me stark naked, and I would have craned my neck around her to see the TV."

You may be feeling a huge sense of relief right about now at the thought that there's a medical issue at play. It means that there's a reason for how he's acting and that it's not personal. He doesn't have some huge dark secret and he's not trying to hurt you.

# What to Expect at This Point

- *You and your husband are both confused and frustrated with what's going on in your marriage.*
- *You probably find yourself arguing a lot and you likely feel disconnected from each other.*
- *You've talked about the situation so often that he has put up shields and refuses to talk about it anymore.*

# Action Steps

- *Put away the sharp implements; you're not going to need them. Not until Chapter 10, anyway.*
- *Realize that you're not some kind of a freak for wanting a healthy sex life with your husband.*
- *Understand that there's a reason for your husband's missing libido.*
- *Recognize that low testosterone kills a guy's sex drive and his ability to live a full life.*
- *Take the Low T Quiz in this chapter and see if it matches up with what's going on in your house.*

*"The light's green," I said.*

*My husband still hesitated.*

*"What's the matter?" I asked.*

*"We turn left, right?" he asked.*

*"What? Yes, turn left," I responded, my voice short and irritated.*

*"We've been to the mall a thousand times," I said, trying to control the tone of my voice. "How can you not know which way to turn? I am so tired of you wanting me to do all the thinking for you."*

*"You know I'm not good with directions," he replied quietly.*

When I first met my husband, he could get anywhere. He frequently travelled for his job and navigated strange cities with ease. I couldn't understand what was going on with him. It felt like he wanted me to be his mother and do all the thinking and planning for both of us.

I hated how sharp I had been with him lately but he was driving me insane! We had lived in the same house for more than ten years, but he had started asking me how to get to places he had driven to a million times. It was like his brain had simply stopped working. I was starting to worry about him. His lack of focus just didn't seem normal to me.

# Chapter 2
# Is It Low T?
## *How Do You Know For Sure?*

Okay, your husband has quite a few low testosterone symptoms, but how do you find out for sure if it's low T? It's surprisingly simple really. The quick and dirty solution to solving the mystery is a blood test.

In this chapter, I'll give you the quickest, most convenient ways to go about getting that testosterone level you need in order to move on to the next step.

## Initial Labs

The first thing that needs to happen is to have him actually get the lab work done. Many men are reluctant to take this step, and you may find that your husband is no exception. There are three common obstacles that get in the way of him getting his lab work done:

- *Concerns about how to actually go about it*
- *Concerns about cost*
- *Concerns about what the results will show (especially intimidating for the guy)*

The first two obstacles are fairly simple to overcome and we'll cover them in this chapter. The last obstacle takes a bit more effort; we'll get to it in the next chapter.

## Walk-In Lab

He can get a simple blood test at one of the many walk-in labs around the country. Some labs require a doctor's orders, but many do not. Do a quick google search of 'walk-in labs, no doctor orders' + your zip code. These labs are fairly cheap and often you don't even have to make an appointment. For example, at one walk-in lab in my area, you can test total testosterone for $45 without a doctor's orders.

For now, all he's going to need is his total testosterone result. If that turns up low, there will be other tests to run, but total T is enough for now.

## Primary Care Doctor

If you can't find a walk-in lab in your area that doesn't require a doctor's orders, your husband can also go to his primary care doctor and ask him to write a lab requisition. While this may prove to be cheaper than a walk-in lab depending on how your insurance works, it can also be fraught with problems.

While we'll talk about this in more detail in the next chapter, it's important to note that a lot of guys resist going to see a doctor. One thing that stands in their way is that it's tough enough for them to admit to themselves that they have low T symptoms, let alone describe

> *2 days from now, you could know for sure whether your husband is dealing with low T.*

those symptoms to a doctor. It tends to be embarrassing and intimidating to them. So they end up talking about hockey scores instead.

Another roadblock is that unless they have specialized training in hormones, general practitioners normally don't know much about testosterone and may actively try to dissuade your husband from checking out his levels. I've seen that one happen fairly often. Your guy finally manages to drag himself to the doctor to check his levels only to be told that he's much too young to worry about low testosterone. Of course, this is exactly what he wants to hear, so he heaves a sigh of relief and skips home with no lab work, telling you that the doctor says there's nothing wrong with him and this must all be in your head. At that point, you have a better chance of winning the lottery than getting him back to a doctor.

> *Low T is also called 'hypogonadism'.*
>
> *Hypo = Low or Below Normal*
> *Gonads = Testes or ovaries*

## Just Get That First Test

The goal is to get that initial blood test done the quickest, easiest way possible. Set it up whichever way you think has the best chance of getting your husband there. The easier and more streamlined you can keep the process, the better chance of getting him on-board. You simply need the total testosterone level in order to know if this is even a thing.

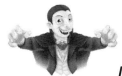

### *I Vant to Suck Your Blood*

*If you are a 'hard stick' as I am ... ie it's tough to draw blood from you ... here are a few tips I've picked up along the way:*

*Hydrate well the day before your blood draw.*

*About an hour before your lab work, put a warming pack on the area from which they'll draw blood.*

*If it's cold weather, make sure to wear warm clothes to keep your veins dilated. Wrapping a blanket around you is helpful.*

*Use some lidocaine cream to numb the area if you'd like.*

*Do some push-ups immediately before the blood draw to dilate veins. Try to do it before the technician walks into the room; otherwise, they'll think you're nuts.*

*Remember to take a deep breath to facilitate blood flow after the technician inserts the needle.*

## Normal Is Not Optimal

Getting the blood test done doesn't do much good if you don't know how to interpret the results. One thing that derails a lot of people is that they assume that a 'normal' T level is a good T level. Let's talk a little bit about what a 'normal' T level means.

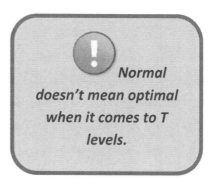

*Normal doesn't mean optimal when it comes to T levels.*

US labs typically measure testosterone in nanograms per deciliter (ng/ dL). Most of them consider anything between 348 and 1197 ng/dL 'normal' when it comes to testosterone, although reference ranges can vary slightly between labs.

The problem with this is that those so-called normal levels encompass a vast variety of men who have tested at that particular lab. The numbers don't take into account a man's age or fitness level. The levels in the reference ranges encompass guys in their 20's … and guys in their 80's! Skinny guys … and fat guys. Guys who are fit … and guys who are not. Your husband's level may be normal … for an 80-year-old man in bad shape! This obviously doesn't make a lot of sense.

A common scenario that I've seen played out over and over again is that a guy (or his wife) suspects he has low T and he finally goes to his primary care office to get it tested. The primary care doc reluctantly writes the lab order and when it comes back at, say 348ng/dL, the doctor says, "Your testosterone is normal." What this means is that a lot of guys go home from their doctor's office feeling like hypochondriacs. At this point, they don't know what else to do so they drop the subject and do nothing. This means they don't get the help they need and nothing gets any better.

Table 1 breaks down testosterone levels by age. Your husband can actually have *half as much testosterone* as he did when he was 20, and still be considered 'normal'. But there is nothing normal about how he feels at this level!

| Age | Total T (ng/dL) | Free T (ng/dL) |
|---|---|---|
| 25-34 | 616 | 12.3 |
| 35-44 | 667 | 10.3 |
| 45-54 | 606 | 9.1 |
| 55-64 | 562 | 8.3 |
| 65-74 | 523 | 6.9 |
| 75-84 | 470 | 6.0 |
| 85-100 | 376 | 5.4 |

Table 1    **Source:** *Androgens and the Aging Male.* Ed. Bjorn Oddens and Alex Vermeulen. New York: The Parthenon Publishing Group Inc., 1996. Print.

Something to remember is that charts are broken down by percentiles. In a reference range of 348-1197ng/dL, for example; 348 is in the **bottom 10th percentile** of the range and 1197 is in the **top 10th percentile**. All of the numbers in between are reported as 'normal'. This is a huge span, however! Certainly the guy in the 10th percentile doesn't feel anywhere near as well as the guy in the 90th percentile. A guy can be in the 10th percentile on the chart and be considered 'normal'. But he's still lower than 90% of other men. Your husband really doesn't want to be in the 10th percentile for a hormone as vital as testosterone.

## A Tale of Two T Levels

Another thing to keep in mind when determining optimal testosterone levels is that we normally don't know a man's baseline level. Here's what I mean. Let's take a look at Alex and Jason, both 21 years old, both in their prime. Their libido and energy levels are high, they build muscle easily, they're active, motivated and have a zest for life. Their testosterone levels, whatever they may be, are exactly where they need to be. They get a baseline drawn and it turns out that Alex' total testosterone level is 900ng/dL, while Jason's is 700. That's a 200 point span, and yet based on how they feel, their testosterone levels are right *for them.*

Twenty years later, both Alex's level and Jason's level have fallen to 600. Same testosterone level, and yet Alex is experiencing low T symptoms while Jason is not. Jason's level has only fallen by 100 points, while Alex' level has fallen a whopping 300 points! Obviously, while the new level is fine for Jason, it's having an enormous negative impact on Alex.

Because we don't check T levels as part of a regular physical, a guy doesn't have any baseline to measure against. He can't look back to when he was on top of the world, and say, "Oh, that was when my T level was at 800. That's the magic number." This is what contributes to the confusion over what an optimal testosterone level is, and it's why it is so important to look not only at lab numbers, but also at symptoms.

Testosterone levels in and of themselves don't tell the full story. Optimal levels are specific to each man. It's not a one-size-fits-all situation. The level at which one man feels absolutely wonderful can be too low for another man. I've seen guys who feel just fine at 700ng/dL, whereas other guys need to be at 800-850ng/dL to feel their best. Experience does show, however, that most guys need to be at least over 500ng/dL in order to feel good, and most men feel their best when they're somewhere in the upper third of the reference range.

## You're Just Getting Older

One thing I hear a lot is that it's 'natural' for testosterone levels to decline in men as they get older and that no one can expect to stay young forever. This is quite true; testosterone levels peak when a man reaches his late teens, stay mostly stable during his 20's and 30's and then begin to decline steadily as he hits his 40's, usually by a percent or two per year. By middle age, most men's testosterone levels will be significantly lower than the peak level they experienced in their late teens to early 20's.

While it's natural for a man's testosterone level to decline somewhat with age, you could also say that it's natural for your vision to decline with age. As we hit middle age, most of us experience a significant change in our reading vision to the extent that eventually we can no longer read a book without reading glasses. From that standpoint, it's 'natural' to not be able to read once you're in your 40's. If we let nature follow its course, those of you who are over 40 would most likely not be able to read the words on this page. We don't say,

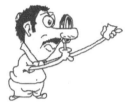

"Hey, you're just getting older. Tough luck." Of course not, that would be ridiculous.

"I'm sorry, Mr. Smith. Your eyesight is getting worse because you're getting older. Just go out and buy yourself a magnifying glass so you can keep reading. Or better yet, I've got these stretches that will make your arms longer so you can hold the book out further."

Just as it's natural to lose your reading vision as you get older, it's also natural for your man's T levels to decrease with age. What's not natural is to pretend that it's not a problem and to refrain from correcting it if possible. Both conditions are treatable and need to be addressed in order to retain quality of life.

## Nature Wants to Kill You!

When people say that it's 'natural' for T levels to decline with age, that this is what Nature intended, my response is that **Nature wants to kill you!** Think about it; Nature is not kind. Nature sends all sorts of natural disasters and diseases raining down upon our heads. Nature is not necessarily your friend. Once you are past the age to produce and raise offspring to survival, Nature is done with you. You've done your job, you've fulfilled your purpose, and Nature starts turning off the tap on the hormones vital to your continued health and well-being. You can either choose to accept that slow decline or actively work to combat the downward slide.

John is a big, burly, 'man's man'. Loves to hunt, hike, and go four-wheeling. He's always been a 'take-no-prisoners' kind of guy ... up until the last few years, that is.

Here's his description of what his life felt like when his levels were 'normal', specifically 381ng/dL.

*"My overall health is good, although I am on meds for high blood pressure. I still need to lose a few pounds and I've got a problem with a lack of energy. I've had issues with ED for a few years now. My doctor said that medically everything is fine, so I guess it's all in my head.*

*We had great sex for most of our marriage. Sometimes sex was the only thing that held us together. Now that that's gone, we just aren't as connected. The past couple of years have been very frustrating. I pretty much lost my desire for sex so that's created a lot of tension. Sex became more work than fun so it just added pressure to the whole act. And I never know when my equipment is going to stop working. It's hard to make myself start something when I don't know if things are going to work.*

*Right now, my attitude drains me. I've been in a kind of rut and can't pull myself out of it. I guess I'm at a mid-life crisis. I'm just not sure what to do with the rest of my life. Nothing is fun anymore. I have issues with depression that I deal with by trying to stay busy.*

*I'm not too excited about much of anything right now. I usually love being outside in nature, but haven't made time for that in a while. Seems like all I do is watch TV anymore. I guess I've lost my desire for heading out these days.*

> *There's a long list of things I need to do around the house, but I can't seem to find the energy or desire to complete them. I need to just suck it up and get some things done. I've always been a 'get her done' kind of guy. I don't know what happened to me."*
>
> *--John, 49, Operations Manager*

To see this big, strong guy reduced to such a shadow of his former self was heartbreaking. But it was so rewarding to watch him come back to life as he got his testosterone up to optimal levels. His 'sweet spot' turned out to be about 800ng/dL. John is now back to his energetic, boisterous self, busily making plans for the second half of his life. He is a force to be reckoned with!

After some ups and downs, he and his wife got back to the passionate, satisfying sex life they had always enjoyed. I thoroughly enjoyed working with them; my only regret is that they had to struggle for so many years before they found their answers.

## Next Step

Now that you understand that normal is not necessarily optimal when it comes to testosterone, you're ready to move on to the next step. You already have a good idea of what his symptoms are, now all you need is his actual number.

That sounds simple in theory, but as I mentioned at the beginning of the chapter, for some of you, getting your husband to that lab is going to be a struggle. If your husband is resistant to the idea of addressing his low testosterone, the next chapter is for you.

# What to Expect at this Point

- *You are feeling your first flickers of hope that your marriage can actually get better.*

- *You feel like the puzzle pieces are finally falling into place, and his behavior is starting to make sense to you.*
- *You'd rather get a root canal than bring this up with your husband, but you can feel your resolve growing.*

# Action Steps

- *Figure out where your husband can get his testosterone tested, and decide if your primary care doctor or a walk-in lab is the best option.*
- *Go ahead and ask your husband to get his testosterone tested, keeping in mind that his response will not be enthusiastic.*
- *If your husband is reluctant to do the initial labs, keep your cool. We'll cover your options in the next chapter.*

# Chapter 3
# The Low T Script
*Knowing What to Expect*

Everything you've read up until now has you convinced that low T may be the culprit in your marriage, and you're ready to move to the next step.

 In this chapter, we'll focus on some common emotions and obstacles that can derail your progress and the steps you need to take in order to move past them.

You may have thought that it would be a fairly simple matter to rule low T in or out with a blood test, but you're hitting some snags when you bring it up to your husband. You may be feeling puzzled and frustrated by his reaction because you don't understand why he's making it such a big deal.

While this is all new and strange to you, low T marriages actually tend to follow a standard script. The emotions and reactions involved are fairly predictable, and knowing the pitfalls ahead of time can make the process go more smoothly. Other couples have gone through this rollercoaster and survived the ride and so can you!

## Both of You Start Out in Denial

A typical scenario in a low T marriage is that the husband is initially in complete denial that there is a problem. The wife gets more and more frustrated with the situation and does a lot of talking about the problem with her husband, whereupon he becomes angry and defensive about the situation and puts up shields to protect himself.

Interestingly enough, quite often the wife starts off in denial as well, although her denial takes a slightly different form. While her husband flat out denies there's a problem at all, the wife fully recognizes that there's an issue; however, she is often reluctant to accept the fact that the cause of the problem may be a medical issue. Thinking that her husband has a medical issue is a scary thought to her because she's used to thinking of him as invulnerable. He, in turn, is used to being able to solve his problems on his own without help, so this is a fundamental paradigm change and difficult for both of them to accept.

By the time the wife goes searching for answers, though, the situation is bad enough that she is willing to put her denial aside in order to get the help they need. Her husband, on the other hand, is usually not quite there yet and because of this, a lot of anger builds up over his reluctance to address the problem.

The relationship has usually deteriorated by this point, with both partners entrenched in their positions. A big part of moving forward is defusing the emotion attached to the problem, and looking at it as a puzzle to be solved. One step toward doing this is simply understanding *why* he reacts as he does.

# Denial is Normal

Your man seems to be in complete denial that there's a problem. It's important to realize that this is quite *normal*. I've never seen a guy who was thrilled to go get his testosterone tested. Some guys are more than reluctant; they're completely resistant. So yes, your husband is probably going to kick and scream about getting his levels tested, but it is what it is. It's simply something you need to work through.

This is how Tom felt about getting his testosterone checked:

*I just don't want to have to try to convince my doctor to check my T levels. I'd have to go over all my symptoms and he might tell me that I'm depressed or some shit like that and try to get me on some crazy anti-depressants.*

*I don't need anyone telling me to jump through their stupid hoops just to get my hormones tested."*

*--Tom, 46, Medical Services*

And Tony:

*"The thing that made me avoid getting lab work was my burning fear of doctors. Sounds stupid, but I waited years because of it."*

—*Tony, 36, IT Technician*

# It's Not Personal

If your guy is dragging his heels, understand it's not personal. While you may feel that the reason he won't address the low T is that he doesn't care about you or the marriage, it actually has nothing to do with you at all. It's about his gut-wrenching fear that there's something 'wrong' with him. Something he can't solve on his own. You think of the situation as being 'just hormones', what's the big deal; he sees your insistence on addressing the issue as an attack on his manhood.

While you may be frustrated and angry with him right now, the key is to put aside those feelings for the moment and keep your cool. Think about it like a traffic jam; you didn't cause it and you couldn't prevent it, you simply have to navigate through it.

# He Hates Dealing with Medical Stuff

Another thing that holds him back is that he hates dealing with medical stuff and the accompanying costs. I frequently see this reaction with men. Of course, that doesn't make him a unique snowflake; most of us hate to deal with doctor's visits and medical stuff and it's normal to be nervous about lab work. While you're probably not thrilled about this whole thing either, the difference is that you're not in that Low T fog and so you are motivated to move past your hesitations in order to fix the problem.

# He's Worried He's Broken

And now we come to the crux of the issue. While it's true that he's probably intimidated by medical stuff and he may have some concerns about what this will cost him, the biggest blockage to him getting that lab work done is *fear.* Specifically, his fear about what the results will show. No man enjoys having his masculinity questioned, and that's probably how your husband is going to feel when you bring up the possibility that his testosterone levels may be low. Brace yourself, this is going to hit him like a punch in the gut. While you may feel relieved to think that you've found some clues to the mystery of the missing libido, I can promise you

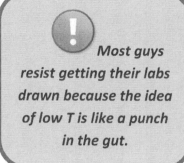

*Most guys resist getting their labs drawn because the idea of low T is like a punch in the gut.*

that your husband isn't going to feel the same way.

Why do so many men react this way? Why do they resist getting their T levels checked to see what's going on? Why are they willing to sacrifice their marriage in order to save their masculine pride?

What you need to realize is that from the time they hit puberty, men identify themselves by their masculinity. They compare themselves to other men. He's bigger, I'm smaller. I'm taller, he's shorter. I'm stronger, he's weaker. They compare muscles, amount of hair, size of penis, and how far they can kick a ball. This is just what guys *do.* There's a huge sense of competition amongst men to be manly. The idea that he's low on the very hormone responsible for masculinity is a bitter pill for your husband to swallow. It strikes at his idea of who he is as a man.

The reason he puts off getting it tested is that he dreads finding out that there's a problem. It's kind of like when you put off doing your breast exam in the shower. You know you should, but then you think, "Wait, I've got that wedding to go to next weekend. If I find a lump, I'll be all depressed and anxious. I don't want to ruin the wedding; I'll just wait until after that." Or you get ready to do the exam, but then you think, "Oh wait, it's a Friday. If I find a lump today, I'll have to wait for the whole weekend before I can get it checked out on Monday. No point in ruining the weekend, I'll wait for Monday."

We all tend to delay doing the stuff that scares us. No one wants to find out that there's a problem. In the same way that you're terrified of finding a lump in your breast, your husband is afraid of discovering that his testosterone levels are low. It's *normal* for him to want to avoid this. Just be firm and loving and hold your ground.

## Real Life Reactions

To give you an idea of what fears may be going through your husband's head, here are some real life reactions from men who discovered that their testosterone levels were low:

*"I used to think I could take care of anything myself and I didn't need any damned doctor to tell me what's wrong with me.*

*When I realized that my testosterone levels were low, I was forced to realize that I'm not as young or indestructible as I used to be, and it was tough to admit. Testosterone is the very essence of masculinity. How can I be a man if mine is low?*

*To think that I'm not as manly as I was … and to go to the doctor and actually have another man tell me that … well, that's just really hard to get past."*

*– Eric, 48, Sound Technician*

*"If my wife came to me and suggested I get my T checked, I'd be insulted and defensive and likely hurt. If she points it out, it means that it is a big deal. It means I can't ignore it anymore and makes me realize that it's a huge damned deal. I really don't want to face that.*

*I'm embarrassed to discuss how my junk is not working and how I have little interest in sex to a male doctor my age who might be judging. I don't want to be the guy who says, 'I need a pill to fix this.' "*

*Plus, I should have healthy testosterone if I'm a man! I feel like I'm saying, 'I'm not a man. Do you have a pill that can change that?' "*

*—Mark, 42, Finance Manager*

Understand that this is a minefield for a guy. When your husband objects to getting his testosterone tested, it may feel like he doesn't care enough to fix the marriage. Give him time. This is really tough for him. Try to stay calm and rational. Emphasize to him that it's simply something that needs to be ruled out.

## Let Go of the Anger

I've devoted a lot of time to what's driving your husband's reluctance to address this issue in the hope that once you understand what's going on, you will be able to release some of the anger that's been building in you.

If your marriage has been struggling for a while, and particularly if your husband has refused to work with you on finding a solution, you're probably feeling really angry with him. This is completely *normal*.

> *While it's normal to feel angry over your situation, anger only slows down your progress.*

It's normal to be frustrated with a husband who has lost his motivation and is no fun to be around. It's normal to be angry when he rejects you. It's normal to feel like life is passing you by.

But the anger isn't helping; in fact, it's making the situation worse. Your anger is pitting the two of you against each other and making it more difficult to move ahead to a resolution. How do you stop feeling so angry?

The first step is to understand that it's not your husband's fault. If his testosterone levels are low, he is dealing with a medical issue currently out of his control. This will take you part of the way to letting go of the anger.

The next step is to get proactive about finding a solution. One reason you feel resentful is that you haven't had any control over what is happening in your marriage. Anger is a normal reaction to feeling powerless. Once you understand what's going on and what you need to do to fix it, you will find that much of your anger dissipates.

The last part to letting go of the anger is getting your sex life back on track, but that happens a bit later in the process.

## Stop Worrying that You're Not Attractive

In addition to anger, another blockage to moving on to a solution is that most women with low drive husbands start doubting their own attractiveness. If your husband has frequently rejected you for sex, your self-esteem has probably taken a real hit. You're starting to doubt your own attractiveness, maybe worrying a little about that extra ten pounds that hasn't come off since the last baby or thinking that you're getting too old to attract your husband.

> **No matter how attractive you are, when your husband's T levels decline, his libido usually does, too.**

I had all those same doubts when my marriage was in the low T fog and my husband not only didn't initiate, he actively *avoided* sex. It was hard for me not to take it personally, but the truth was that it didn't have anything to do with me. It wasn't some deep, complicated issue with our marriage. We didn't need therapy, we didn't need to explore our childhood issues, and we didn't need to have deep discussions about our sex life. What we needed was **hormones**.

Most of us assume that the problem must somehow be our fault. "Why doesn't he seem interested in me physically?" is a reoccurring question that haunts the wife. She has this list that runs through her head. "Am I too fat? Am I out of shape? Maybe I'm boring. Or too critical. I do criticize him a lot. Maybe my boobs are too small, they're definitely droopier than they used to be." And on and on. The wife's diminished confidence is one of the more heartbreaking side effects of being with a man who has lost his sex drive.

Here's Teresa's account of what she did to regain her husband's interest:

> *"My husband lost interest in sex and stopped initiating. I would initiate about once every six weeks when I finally couldn't wait any longer. It would take him 20-30 minutes to get to an orgasm, and every once in a while, he would lose his erection.*
>
> *I thought it must be that I was ugly and he couldn't get aroused, so I had a boob job. I've never been very big, and I know he likes big breasts. I think I look great now; however, it didn't help the problem. I thought it was me, but now I'm not so sure.*
>
> *This is destroying our marriage because I can't get over his lack of sexual desire for me. Every time I bring up the problem, he turns it back on me and I can't get a straight answer. This is ripping me apart emotionally. I need help! If we don't figure this out, I cannot stay with this guy."*
>
> *-- Teresa, 41, Account Manager*

Months later, upon him finally checking his testosterone levels, it turned out that her husband had the testosterone levels of that 80-year-old man I talked about! All the angst she went through was for nothing. He had a *medical issue* that had nothing to do with whether she was attractive or not.

Here's what Ben had to say on the matter:

> *"I don't know what it is. I love my wife, she's in good shape; I still think she's attractive, but I just don't have the same drive. I initiate occasionally, but it's more like something I know I should do rather than that 'I've got to have her' feeling it used to be."*
>
> *—Ben, 37, Teacher*

That lets you hear it from both the husband and wife's perspective. So by all means, work out and get fit and make the most of your appearance but understand that your husband's lack of sex drive most likely has absolutely nothing at all to do with you. If he has low testosterone, neither of you are doing anything wrong; there's simply a medical issue that needs correcting.

# Reframe the Issue

All right. You're starting to understand that the emotions you've been feeling, while normal, have actually worked against finding a solution to the problem. There's been a lot of anger and resentment leading up to this point. There may even have been some yelling matches somewhere along the way where both of you have thrown around insults and accusations at each other. Where do you go from here?

With your new knowledge, it's time to reframe the discussion. It's not about who's right and who's wrong; it's about him dealing with a possible medical problem. No different than getting your dentist to check out a sore tooth.

You need to get calm and rational about all this. You have a mystery that has an answer and your goal is to find that answer. It's not about making your husband the bad guy and it's not about assigning blame. What you need to do is to let your husband know that you love him and that you're on his team; together you will find the answers to repair your marriage. Your anger, resentment, and doubts about yourself simply get in the way of finding those answers, so you need to let all of that go. We're going to tackle this problem step by step together.

# Stop Talking to Him About Sex

One of the most important things you need to do is to stop talking to him about sex. I'll be honest, this is a tough one. It's really hard to stop talking about something that's so important to you. But look at it this way … you've had a million conversations with him about why he doesn't want sex anymore, and it hasn't helped. He never gives the same answer twice and you feel like you're going crazy. Every conversation you have increases the knot of tension between the two of you. You feel your anxiety start to rise every evening, wondering if this is going to be the night he finally initiates. You can keep it together for a while, but when too many nights go by without him initiating, you end up exploding.

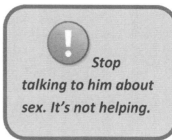

*Stop talking to him about sex. It's not helping.*

Unfortunately, every time you talk to him about his lack of sex drive, it simply makes him feel more damaged than he already does. Look, he *knows* that something's wrong. He may pretend that it's you who has unrealistic expectations … "Honey, married couples don't have sex that often. I don't know *any* other couples who have a lot of sex. Why can't you be happy with once every couple of weeks?" … but he *knows* that there's an issue.

*"She woke me up a little past five this morning. At first, I couldn't figure out what she wanted. Then it dawned on me that duh, she wanted sex.*

*My initial response was to pretend to still be sleeping because lately sex just doesn't feel all that great. Or at least not great enough to give up sleep for.*

*I wish she would give it a rest with always wanting sex."*

*--Mark, 42, Finance Manager*

In addition to making him feel defensive, the problem with complaining to him about the lack of sex is that it continually frames you as the pursuer, which causes him to want to pull away. We'll get to this later on in the book, but this is also setting you up for more problems later on after you address the medical and start repairing the marriage.

You don't need more talk; you need *action*. The more you talk about the issue, the thicker his shields get. The longer you struggle with this issue, the more resentment builds between the two of you. The two of you need to be on the same team over this issue. It's neither of your fault, you simply have to fix it.

## Stop Feeling Guilty

Your next step is to deal with your feelings of guilt. Because so many men fight the idea of addressing their low T, often the wife is the one who initiates the process. This typically only happens once she's

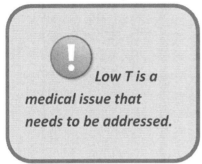

*Low T is a medical issue that needs to be addressed.*

reached the end of her rope. She has put up with … *and* put up with … *and* put up with … until she just can't put up with anymore. By the time she starts searching for answers, she is desperate. She usually feels that she's pushing her husband against his will to do this

*for her*, while he gets no benefit from it. Nothing could be further from the truth.

Right about now, you may be feeling like the meanest woman who ever lived. Your husband is miserable about getting his T levels tested and you are feeling selfish for asking him to do this. What you need to understand is that low testosterone is about much more than just a lack of sex. Low T is associated with a multitude of health issues that are quite damaging to not only a man's health, but also his quality of life.

My husband has thanked me over and over for doing the research about low testosterone and refusing to let it go when he initially resisted. He feels a thousand times better than he did before. He feels younger, stronger and more energetic. His career is more productive, he's a better husband and a more active dad. He works out regularly, practices a martial art and feels so much more like a man than he did when his testosterone levels were low. It's as if he has a new lease on life.

I often talk with men who feel the same way and are thankful that their wives cared enough to persist in finding answers. You are not being selfish in wanting to fix this issue. You love this guy and want him around for a long time. Even more than living a long life, you want him to live a full life and a healthy one. You can't afford to let this issue die. There's too much at stake. Keep that in mind when the going gets tough and you start to feel like you should simply let the whole thing drop.

Here's what Steve says about the wife who held his feet to the fire:

*"Persuading me to go get my T levels checked was the best thing my wife ever did for me. On hormone therapy, I am alive like never before. I actually want sex with my beautiful wife again. Energy is also through the roof!*

*My only regret is the years my wife and I both lost when we could have been enjoying this passion together all along."*
—*Steve, 43, Technician*

Because low T affects cognitive ability and motivation, when your husband is in the low T fog, it's up to you to help him find his way out. In the same way that people dealing with depression don't realize that their symptoms aren't normal, a guy with low testosterone levels is quite often the last person to recognize that there's a problem. That's where you come in. You're the person who knows him best and you will be the first to realize that something is going on with him. It's okay for you to say, "Enough is enough. Either you make the appointment or I will." This is a reasonable expectation, and you need to hold the line on it.

Consider what Sloane Teeple, MD, urologist and author of *"I'm Still Sexy, So What's Wrong with Him?"* had to say:

*"I simply didn't know that my sex drive wasn't where it was supposed to be. The loss of libido had come gradually and both Susan and I had attributed it to the stressors of a high-pressure medical residency. We were wrong." (p. 3)*

If a doctor trained in men's reproductive issues didn't recognize his own low T symptoms, can you really expect your husband to? While it's frustrating to watch your husband stick his head in the sand, it's important that you don't give up on him. He needs you to be his advocate, now more than ever.

## It's Not Just About Sex

Here's some information to bolster your resolve when you start to doubt yourself. Low T has vast health implications for a man quite aside

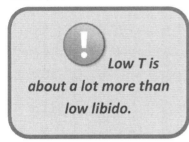

**Low T is about a lot more than low libido.**

from his libido. While a lack of a satisfying sex life may be what initially drove you to look for answers, there's a much bigger picture out there. Once you realize the broader impact low T has on your husband's life, it will become even more important to you

to find out if it's an issue for him.

Even if you had absolutely no interest in ever having a sex life with your husband again, you would still need to understand the impact low testosterone has on his health. After all, no matter how bad things are between the two of you at the moment, you still love this guy and want the best for him. It's important to realize that testosterone is associated with not only how *well* your man lives, but actually how *long* he lives.

Consider that men with low testosterone …

- *Are **four times more likely** to be diagnosed with depression*
- *Are **twice as likely** to die from cardiovascular disease*
- *Have **double** the risk of getting osteoporosis*
- *Have **four times** the risk of developing diabetes*
- *Are much more likely to develop Alzheimer's disease. For every 10-unit increase in testosterone levels, the risk of developing Alzheimer's goes down by **slightly more than 25 percent**.*
- *And the final kicker … Men with low T are **40 percent more likely to die** (during a specific time period) than men with healthy testosterone levels.*

When you start to doubt yourself because he's stressed out about what his lab results will show and you're starting to wonder if you made a mistake in pushing the issue, come back and take another look at these statistics and let them remind you how important it is to resolve this health issue.

# Start Tracking Sex Frequency

Your next step is to track how often you're having sex. Or more accurately, how seldom. It doesn't have to be complicated, just a list of the days you had sex and who initiated.

The reason for tracking sex is that most low drive guys vastly over-estimate the amount of sex they're having and are blind to the fact that there's a problem. This conversation may sound familiar to you:

*"All you ever want to do is watch TV. Why don't you ever want sex anymore?"*

*"What? What are you talking about? We don't have to watch TV if there's something else you'd rather do." (Turns off the TV). "What do you want to do? Do you want to go out or something?"*

*"NO! I want to stay in. As in 'in bed'. What I'm asking is why you never initiate sex."*

*"I don't know why you say that. I initiate sex all the time."*

*"When's the last time we had sex? Do you even know?"*

*"It was like five nights ago, wait, maybe six, because I had that work meeting Wednesday night and I was tired when I got home from that. So it was the night after that, yeah, it must be about six nights ago."*

*"For your information, that work meeting was three weeks ago. We haven't had sex for three weeks!"*

*He looks dumbfounded. "No, that can't be right."*

You feel like killing him and wonder whether he's being purposely obtuse. I can tell you that he's not; this is absolutely typical for a low T guy. Sex simply isn't on his radar. It's like a switch got turned off in his brain and while it feels personal to you, it's not. He really can't help it.

This is why tracking sex is going to help. While he may be able to convince himself that you're exaggerating when you merely *tell* him how much the sex has decreased, he can't deny the facts when you put them in front of him in black and white. This typically hits a guy square in the eyes and he has that 'aha' moment where he finally realizes that something really is off. It puts an end to the 'he said, she said' dynamic that has been fogging the whole issue.

This is how it worked out for one woman:

*"I made a chart of our sexual interactions for the last few months, and showed it to my husband. It showed that we are having sex about every six weeks. I told him that one reason I am freaking out is that I don't want to live in a sexless marriage.*

*He looked absolutely flabbergasted and had tears in his eyes. It's like that chart erased the smokescreen he's been putting up. I felt like a murderer, but something has to give. For the first time, I feel like he actually heard what I'm saying."*

## Initiate 'The Conversation'

Okay, you've made a lot of progress so far. You've let go of the anger and resentment, you've stopped complaining to him about sex, and you've tracked your sex frequency and have proof-in-hand that there's a problem. Now what? How do you actually bring this subject up with him in a loving, tactful way?

While *you* understand that he needs to get that initial lab work done, *he's* dragging his feet; and you can see that it's going to be an uphill battle to get him to that lab. It's going to take a bit of tact to navigate these tricky waters. It's time for ... gulp ... *The Conversation.*

While this isn't going to be a pleasant discussion, there are some things you can do to make it go down a bit easier. You're going to want to start off with a clear statement about the problem in a way that isn't accusatory or derogatory. Pick a time where both of you are relaxed and you're sure there won't be any interruptions. Don't have this conversation when you're feeling hurt or angry at a recent rejection. You want to frame this in a way that's as positive and productive as you can manage.

> *"Honey, there are some things I'm seeing in our marriage that have me concerned."*

Then go on to calmly list your concerns.

> *"I've noticed that you are frequently tired, you're having a tough time losing the extra weight, you're having difficulty remembering things and focusing on things, and your energy levels have dropped."*

Then hand him your sex frequency chart.

> *"I've also noticed that we're not having nearly as much sex as we used to."*

Calm, rational, loving. That's your frame.

> *"I've been reading up on the issue and there are actually a lot of couples going through the same thing we are. From what I'm reading, it seems that low testosterone can cause a lot of the issues we're seeing. I think the first step is to get that checked out. I've done some research and there's a clinic where you can get your levels checked without having to worry about a doctor appointment."*

At this point, you hand him the information about the walk-in lab or the doctor appointment card.

So there you go. That's pretty much it. It's not a conversation you look forward to but it has to happen. Once it's done, you will breathe a huge sigh of relief. Because you will be one step closer to solving the mystery.

## More Real Life Reactions

In an ideal world, your husband would react like this …. "Thank you so much, sweetheart! What a fine and caring wife you are to be concerned. Let me go right now and get my levels checked because that's just how much I love you."

In the real world … not so much. Remember that whole 'punch in the gut' thing? Most husbands really struggle with this conversation. You can assume that he's going to feel defensive and angry.

Here's an example of one husband's reaction when his wife talked to him about getting his T levels checked out:

*"I suggested that he get his testosterone levels checked and he blew a gasket! He made some incredibly hurtful comments and a lot of angry remarks. He told me that it wasn't him that was the problem, it was me. That I should see a psychologist because I am such a sex maniac. I don't think wanting sex more than once a month makes me a nymphomaniac!"*

Be aware that he may throw the problem back on you. "If you were sexier, maybe I would want more sex! It's because you do nothing except nag me about sex. No guy wants it under those circumstances." You've got to ignore all that. It's not your husband talking; it's just his fear.

Stay calm and simply repeat the goal, "You may be right. Low testosterone may not be the issue, but we need to rule it out so that we know what we're dealing with."

Also be prepared for the fact that he may put up a smokescreen for the next few weeks and initiate a lot of sex in an effort to convince you (and himself) that low T isn't the issue. Hey, great. Enjoy the sex. When he eventually runs out of steam because he can't sustain the necessary energy, get him to the lab.

Lori experienced this first hand:

> *"I asked my husband to read the list of low T symptoms and he came up about an hour later and said, 'I have most of the symptoms on there.' I replied, 'Do you think that could be what is affecting your sex drive and why we are having so many problems?' He agreed with me and gave me a huge hug. Then he locked our door, tossed me on the bed and had his way with me.*
>
> *We had sex three times that week and I was excited that maybe the problem was solved, but then he stopped initiating and we haven't had sex since."*
>
> *– Lori, 41, Property Manager*

Now obviously, not all men react negatively to getting their testosterone tested. There are some guys out there who are fine with getting their T levels checked, or at least willing to do it even if they're not thrilled. If you have one of them, you get to skip this chapter and move straight on to the next chapter. But a surprisingly large number of men react quite badly to the suggestion that they get the lab work done, so you need to be prepared for that possibility.

# What to Expect at this Point

- *Your marriage is extremely low energy.*
- *Sex is infrequent and not all that exciting.*
- *Your husband is tired and discouraged.*

- *You feel angry and resentful that your husband has his head in the sand and is dragging his feet.*
- *While you initially hated to think there was a medical problem, you've reached the point of wanting to find answers.*
- *Your worry about whether you're attractive.*
- *You argue frequently, particularly about sex.*
- *The situation gets worse when you ask him to test his levels. He feels emasculated, and may even lash out at you in anger.*
- *He may blame you for the lack of sex.*
- *You may see a temporary uptick in sex as he strives to prove to himself that he's still 'got it'.*

# Action Steps

- *Let go of the anger and start taking action.*
- *Stop worrying about whether you're attractive.*
- *Reframe the issue.*
- *Stop talking to him about sex.*
- *Stop feeling guilty for asking him to get his lab work done.*
- *Understand the health implications of low T and discuss them with your husband.*
- *Track sex frequency.*
- *Initiate a conversation and ask your husband (again) to get his testosterone tested.*
- *Be prepared in case he responds badly, and respond calmly and productively.*

"I'm going for a walk, do you want to come?" I asked.

"No, that's okay," he responded, his eyes never leaving the TV. "I'm feeling pretty tired tonight."

I felt a rising sense of irritation. He was **always** tired. I was tired of him feeling tired. I was taking off the final few pounds of baby weight, but he seemed content to just sit around and watch TV, getting more overweight and out of shape with each passing day.

It was like there was no **bounce** left in him. Where was that spark that had drawn me to him in the first place?

# Chapter 4
# No Laughing Matter
## *Health Implications of Low T*

His lab results are in and *dun...dun...DUHN!* It's Miss Scarlet, with the lead pipe, in the Conservatory. His testosterone levels are 351ng/dL. While this is 'normal', according to the reference range on the lab results, you now know that it's actually normal for an 85-year-old, and this low level is most likely contributing to the symptoms your husband is experiencing.

You finally have a solution to your mystery. Now what? If he's like most guys, your husband looks like all the wind has been taken out of his sails, and you're wondering if you should have just let sleeping dogs lie. He's shocked and discouraged. It's like you can see his manhood shrinking right in front of your eyes. For you, it's a bit scary, but also hopeful. Finally, you have a tangible reason for what's going on in your marriage.

Your husband seems so deflated that you may be second guessing yourself on pursuing the issue of his low testosterone, but there are important medical reasons for doing so which I detail in this chapter.

## How Low is Low?

You already know from Chapter 2 that normal is not optimal, but how do you know if your husband's level of 351ng/dL actually warrants treatment. After all, according to the lab's reference range, it's 'normal'. Understand that this is a judgment call on the part of you and your husband. There's nothing that says that he *has* to treat his testosterone level of 351. In fact, many doctors would tell him that he's just fine at that level.

However, you *know* he's not just fine. You can see the changes that have taken place in him. What I can tell you is that for many men a level of 351 is simply not high enough for them to feel good and have a robust sex drive. In fact, he probably feels somewhat like that 85-year old man who shares the same testosterone level.

I mentioned in Chapter 3 that lower testosterone levels are associated with multiple health problems like cardiovascular disease, diabetes, osteoporosis, Alzheimer's, and depression. Taking a deeper look at the information behind those statistics is eye opening.

## The Heart of the Matter

Coronary heart disease is the leading killer of men in the US, and testosterone levels under 500ng/dL are correlated with a higher risk of cardiovascular problems. In fact, low T is one of the main predictors of whether a man will eventually have cardiovascular problems. The research on this is astounding!

One study followed 2,416 men for five years. Men with the highest testosterone levels had a 30% lower risk of having cardiovascular events (heart attacks, strokes, etc.), while men with the lowest testosterone levels were twice as likely to have cardiovascular disease.

In another study, researchers followed 504 non-smoking men. Men with the highest testosterone levels had a risk reduction of 60-80% of severe aortic atherosclerosis (hardening and narrowing of the arteries-a major risk factor for heart attack and stroke) even after adjusting for age and other risk factors. In addition, lower testosterone levels are associated with high blood pressure, higher LDL (bad) cholesterol and higher triglycerides, all of which are risk factors for cardiovascular problems.

## Diabetes and Insulin Resistance

More than 29 million Americans have diabetes, almost ten percent of the population. By this point, you're not going to be surprised to hear that testosterone plays a key role here as well. Low testosterone levels can actually be used to predict the development of type 2 diabetes. In fact, the association between diabetes and low T is so pronounced that the Endocrine Society recommends that men who have been diagnosed with Diabetes 2 get their testosterone levels checked.

Men whose free testosterone levels are in the lowest third of the reference range are **four times more likely to develop diabetes**. Given that diabetes contributes to high blood pressure and can significantly increase the risk of heart attacks, this is an important statistic and one that doesn't bode well for guys with low testosterone.

# It's In His Bones

We also know that one of the strongest predictors of bone density in an older man is how much testosterone he has circulating in his blood stream. The risk of osteoporosis in men with deficient testosterone levels is **roughly double** that of men with normal levels. Healthy testosterone equals healthy bones

While osteoporosis may seem like some far-off future problem that happens to old people, here's where it gets interesting. Bone loss typically begins in the mid-30's; coincidentally, this is when testosterone levels start to decline in men. Bone loss can manifest quite subtly at first with low-back pain, joint or muscle aches, a loss in height and hunched shoulders, or it may not have any symptoms at all initially. Left unchecked, bone loss goes on to have devastating effects on a man, and it all begins with testosterone.

> *The word 'osteoporosis' comes from Latin and literally means 'porous bones'.*

# Cognitive Function and Alzheimer's Disease

Multiple studies have confirmed the link between low testosterone and Alzheimer's disease. For example, in the Baltimore Longitudinal Study of Aging, researchers followed 574 men, aged 32 – 87, for almost 20 years and found that **for every 10-unit increase in free testosterone levels, the risk of developing Alzheimer's went down by slightly more than 25 percent.**

In addition, testosterone levels are associated with memory and cognitive functions. Am I saying that if your husband starts addressing his low testosterone levels, he will turn into the next Stephen Hawking? Well, no, but I am saying that deficient testosterone levels may be impairing his ability to think and remember, as well as being associated with a higher incidence of Alzheimer's disease.

# Depression

Men with low testosterone are *four times more likely to be diagnosed with depression*, and yet doctors rarely check testosterone levels when a man presents with symptoms of depression.

## LOW TESTOSTERONE AND ALZHEIMER'S DISEASE

In 2010, researchers working with geriatric patients found a correlation in low testosterone levels and a man's risk of getting Alzheimer's disease. Since then, multiple studies have confirmed the link between Alzheimer's and low testosterone.

**"We found that low testosterone did predict a pretty rapid decline in memory and conversion to Alzheimer's, so this opens up the possibility of using testosterone as a potential treatment in males who are having early memory problems."**

-- *John Morley MD, Professor of Gerontology and Director of the Division of Geriatric Medicine at Saint Louis University School of Medicine in Missouri*

The real tragedy is that when a man goes to his doctor for these symptoms, he is often diagnosed with depression and prescribed an anti-depressant with all its attendant side effects, including decreased libido, without ever addressing his low testosterone. What a shame that we don't routinely test men who are struggling with depression for low testosterone *before* prescribing an anti-depressant.

# All-Cause Mortality

By far, the most startling information about low testosterone is its effect on a man's mortality. Multiple studies have shown that men with low testosterone levels are more likely to die sooner than men with healthy testosterone levels, even after controlling for age, weight and other lifestyle factors.

In one long-term study conducted by University of Cambridge gerontologist Kay-Tee Khaw, researchers followed more than 11,000 men aged 40-79 for 10 years. Compared to men with the lowest testosterone levels, men with the highest levels were 41% less likely to die over the next 10 years. That's a pretty amazing finding!

This is not an isolated result. Other studies reveal similar findings. In a study of 794 men aged 50-91 conducted in California, researchers found that men with the lowest testosterone levels were 40% more likely to die over a specified time period than those with higher levels. Again, that is quite startling! What's more, the body of research that bears out similar findings is growing every year.

Consider this finding from *The Journal of Clinical Endocrinology and Metabolism*.

> *"Men whose total testosterone levels were in the lowest quartile (<241 ng/dl) were 40% more likely to die (during the course of the study) than those with higher levels, independent of age, adiposity (fat), and lifestyle."*

Let's take another look at that chart. Does your husband really want to have the testosterone levels of an elderly man?

| Age | Total T (ng/dL) | Free T (ng/dL) |
|---|---|---|
| 25-34 | 616 | 12.3 |
| 35-44 | 667 | 10.3 |
| 45-54 | 606 | 9.1 |
| 55-64 | 562 | 8.3 |
| 65-74 | 523 | 6.9 |
| 75-84 | 470 | 6.0 |
| 85-100 | 376 | 5.4 |

Table 2    **Source:** *Androgens and the Aging Male*. Ed. Bjorn Oddens and Alex Vermeulen. New York: The Parthenon Publishing Group Inc., 1996. Print.

## Feeling Overwhelmed

At this point, your husband is probably reeling a bit, feeling lost and discouraged and finding it difficult to take in all the information he needs to learn. You are his best advocate, and as long as he is in the low T fog, he's going to need your help.

You may also be feeling overwhelmed. It may seem like all this is a heavy burden and you would just like to get back to normal life. Remember that it won't be this way forever. You'll find your way forward, meet the challenge and this will just be a blip on the radar. Once your husband gets back on his feet again, he'll be able take his share of the burden, but for the moment your support is vital.

All of this is new to both of you. It's normal to be anxious when you face the unknown. Let's take some more of the mystery out of it for you. In *Stage Two*, we're going to talk about what testosterone is, what is does, what causes it to drop, and what options are available to bring those levels back up to optimal.

# What to Expect at this Point

- *Your husband feels depressed and discouraged when his low testosterone is confirmed. This is normal, and he'll start feeling better once he understands that there are great options out there for correcting the problem.*

- *You are torn between feeling angry with him that he's dragging his feet on dealing with the problem, guilty over the pressure you're putting on him, and hopeful that there's a solution for the problems in your marriage.*

- *You both will probably feel anxious now that you know the health implications of low T. That's not necessarily a bad thing if it motivates you to act.*

- *Sex is as infrequent as ever; in fact, it actually may be less frequent now that you don't nag him for sex anymore.*

- *Hang in there, this stage won't last forever.*

# Action Steps

- *Understand that you need to be your husband's advocate until he's back on his feet.*

- *Educate yourself and your husband about the health implications of low testosterone.*

# Stage Two

# Finding a Solution

*"What did the doctor say?"* I asked excitedly.

After finally identifying low testosterone as a possible cause of my husband's symptoms and battling to get him to see a doctor, he had finally gone to his appointment. This was the first chance we had found to talk since getting the kids to bed and I was on pins and needles waiting to hear what the doctor had to say.

*"He said that I'm just getting older,"* my husband announced tiredly.

*"What?"* I asked disbelievingly.

*"Yeah, he told me I just needed to diet and exercise some more."*

*"But ...... but did you tell him that you've been dieting and exercising diligently for two* **years** *now? Did you tell him that the weight isn't budging? That you're more tired now than when you started? That you fall asleep all the time and you feel like crap. Did you tell him you think your testosterone levels might be low?"*

I fired questions at him, my voice getting higher and more anxious with each one. I knew I was over-reacting, but my husband's resigned acceptance was making my brain crazy.

*"He told me that testosterone therapy is dangerous and will make my testicles shrink,"* my husband replied.

*"That's IT? That's all he said?"* I asked, my voice raising several decibels as I wanted to throw something.

*"Yeah, that's all he had to say. He said I'm doing pretty well, to watch my cholesterol and he'll see me in a year for my next check-up."*

# Chapter 5
# Testosterone Primer
## *More than You Ever Wanted to Know*

It's important to understand what testosterone is and how it's made in order to understand what's gone wrong with your husband's

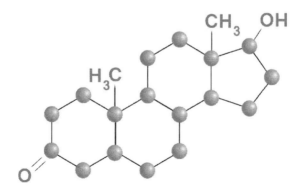

production and what can be done to fix it. In this chapter, I'll talk about the basics of testosterone production and in the next chapter, I'll discuss what can go wrong in the process.

## What is Testosterone?

At its most basic level, testosterone is the feel-good hormone for men. It produces energy, motivation and feelings of well-being. It drives ambition, confidence and libido. It affects lean body mass and ability to build muscle. Testosterone helps a man get and keep firm erections and have strong orgasms. In other words, testosterone is what makes a man feel like ... well, a man.

Here's an illustration of what a testosterone molecule looks like:

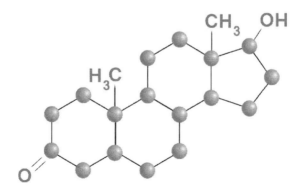

**Testosterone**

Testosterone is a steroid hormone produced mainly by a man's **testicles (gonads)**, with much smaller amounts produced by the adrenal glands. We hear the words 'hormone' and 'steroid' frequently, but what exactly do those words mean?

A **hormone** is a chemical produced in your body that is transported to different areas via the bloodstream where it produces different types of responses. For example, insulin is a hormone produced in the pancreas that is moved throughout the body, controlling how your cells utilize glucose. Estrogen is a hormone that stimulates breast development and is produced mainly by a woman's ovaries. Testosterone is a hormone that is produced by the testicles and then travels through the bloodstream to various tissues and organs.

## 'Steroid' Is Not a Four-Letter Word

When you hear the word 'steroid', you may think of bodybuilders and 'roid rage'; however, everyone produces steroids 24/7. That's right; you are a steroid user! We all are. The difference is that our bodies produce natural steroids and not the synthetic steroids that you think of when you see bodybuilders with huge muscles. A *steroid* is simply an organic compound with a particular molecular structure. Each of us produces multiple types of steroid hormones such as testosterone, estrogen, cortisol and progesterone. Without them, you couldn't survive.

> **Both men and women produce multiple steroid hormones.**

The difference between bodybuilders who abuse steroids and regular guys who use testosterone replacement is huge. A bodybuilder who is using 'roids' is using testosterone-like compounds at levels that are much higher than normal to get results that he couldn't normally achieve. A guy with low T is simply replacing the testosterone his body is no longer producing in order to get back to healthy levels. Those are two very different propositions.

> *A woman's body also produces testosterone, although at much lower levels -- about a tenth as much as a man's.*

# How Testosterone Is Made

A man's body produces testosterone in a multi-step process that involves the testes (gonads) and the hypothalamus and pituitary glands. Together they form the **HPG (Hypothalamus-Pituitary-Gonadal) axis**. These glands work together in a complex series of interactions and feedback loops to keep a man's testosterone at a healthy level. Dysfunction in any of the three components can cause problems with testosterone production. How you treat low T depends on where the dysfunction occurs.

Here's how it works. It starts with the hypothalamus gland, a tiny gland in your brain right above your brain stem. The hypothalamus produces **gonadotropin-releasing hormone (GnRH)**, and sends it to the pituitary gland, a pea-sized structure right below the hypothalamus. This stimulates the pituitary to produce two hormones - **luteinizing hormone (LH)** and **follicle stimulating hormone (FSH).**

LH regulates the production of testosterone and FSH regulates the production of sperm. Both LH and FSH, after being produced by the pituitary, travel through the blood stream to the testes to stimulate the production of testosterone and sperm. While the testicles are what produce testosterone, it's actually the hypothalamus and pituitary that tell the testicles when and how much to produce.

Then through a complex, multi-step process, LH stimulates the **Leydig cells** in a man's testicles to convert cholesterol into testosterone. Once testosterone is produced, it travels through the bloodstream to exert its beneficial effects on the various tissues and organs that are equipped with testosterone receptors. These include bone, fat and muscle cells, the heart and brain, the sex organs and the vocal cords, to name a few.

That's a lot of information to take in, so take a look at the illustration below to get a visual picture of what's going on.

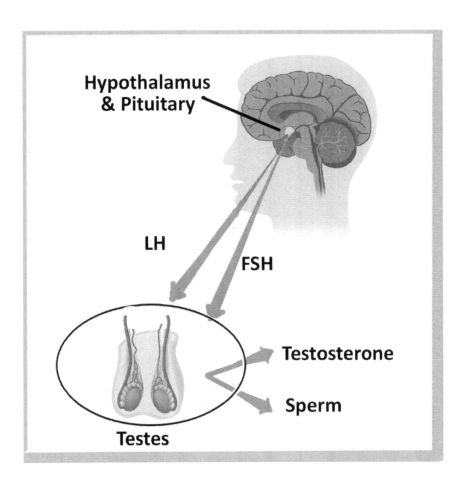

That's pretty much the condensed version of testosterone production, but it will give you enough to go on for the moment. In the next chapter, we'll move on to what can go wrong in the process, and how you can correct it.

# What to Expect at this Point

- *You both may feel overwhelmed at all there is to learn about low testosterone and treatment options.*
- *You may also be feeling relieved at this point that there's a clearly identifiable reason for what's going on.*

# Action Steps

- *Gain a basic understanding of how the body produces testosterone so that you can understand treatment options.*
- *Recognize that testosterone treatment is different than steroid abuse.*

*"Honey, wake up."*

*"What?" he said groggily.*

*"Wake **up**!" I repeated, "The alarm's gone off four times now."*

*I turned back over, not wanting to start the day off on a sour note. The baby had gotten me up three times last night and I was exhausted. Why couldn't my husband just get up when the alarm went off instead of hitting the snooze over and over again until it finally woke me up?*

*It wasn't like he wasn't getting enough sleep. He had fallen asleep at 8:30 last night on the sofa until I had woken him up to go to bed. Why was it that I was the one who was up several times a night nursing a baby, but he was the one who was tired all the time?*

*Between the baby getting me up and my husband's snoring keeping me up, I felt bone-tired.*


No matter how much sleep my husband got, he was always tired. He snored a lot. I started listening and realized that he actually stopped breathing sometimes. He fell asleep anytime he sat down with the kids and sometimes even in church. I just couldn't understand what had happened to that high energy, always-on-the-go man I had married!

Many years and many doctors later, we were to find that he had sleep apnea, which is inextricably linked to low testosterone. How I wish I had known then what I know now! We could have avoided so much angst.

# Chapter 6
# The Usual Suspects
## *Factors that Contribute to Low T*

Now that you understand the basics of testosterone production, let's look at where it may have gone off-track for your husband.

There are multiple factors that can disrupt testosterone production in a man's body, some that are controllable by lifestyle choices and others that are not. Some can be detected through blood work or physical examination while others cannot.

In a system as complex as testosterone production, you can't always figure out where things have run amok. You can try your best to isolate the problem, but sometimes at the end of the day all you know is that his body isn't making enough testosterone. In those cases, while you can replace the missing testosterone, you simply can't correct the root causes. Hopefully, one day medical science will be far enough along to accurately identify causes of low testosterone more consistently but we're not there yet.

In this way, low T is no different from hypothyroidism or juvenile diabetes. A doctor can't always definitively tell you why your thyroid or your pancreas went awry. All they can do is to replace the missing thyroid hormone or the missing insulin your body is no longer making.

This was the case for my husband. Even though his doctor ran multiple labs to find the core cause of his low testosterone production, we never got any clear answers. My husband ended up simply replacing the missing testosterone with an external source. While it would have been nice to actually find and fix the root cause, it's not the end of the world. Even though he'll never know what caused his T levels to decrease, he still feels a thousand percent better on T therapy than off it!

Understanding that many - maybe most - men are never able to find out precisely why their testosterone production went wrong, let's look at some factors that *can* be ruled out. An experienced hormone replacement specialist will try to eliminate the following factors before suggesting treatment options. If possible, they will work with your husband to correct any underlying causes of low T.

Increased ferritin (iron), elevated prolactin, and elevated estrogen can all cause problems with T levels. Varicoceles are varicose veins in the testes and can lower testosterone production.

Lifestyle also factors into testosterone levels. Heavy alcohol use, certain meds and drugs, and obesity can all play a role. Sleep apnea normally lowers testosterone production, as do nutritional deficiencies, diabetes and thyroid dysfunction. If there is an identifiable issue like one of those listed above, correcting it will quite often correct testosterone production. Table 3 shows different causes of low T and methods of identifying them.

## Methods of Identifying Factors Associated with Lower T Levels

| Determined by Lab Work | Determined by Physical Exam | Determined by Medical History |
|---|---|---|
| • Elevated ferritin | • Varicoceles & other abnormalities | • Drug Use or Other Meds |
| • Elevated estrogen | • Obesity | • Alcohol Use |
| • Elevated prolactin | • Sleep apnea | • Genetic conditions |
| • Nutritional deficiencies | | |
| • Diabetes | | |
| • Thyroid problems | | |

Table 3

In many and probably most cases, though, none of these factors are issues. At that point, the doctor may suggest other labs in order to figure out where the problem may be occurring.

# All in Your Head or Further South?

As we talked about in the previous chapter, there are three major organs and glands involved in testosterone production; the testicles and the hypothalamus and pituitary glands. Problems in any of these areas can cause problems with T production.

There are three main categories of hypogonadism; primary, secondary and combination. (Remember that hypogonadism is another term for low T.) If your husband's problem originates in his testes, then he's dealing with *primary hypogonadism*. If, on the other hand, the problem originates in his hypothalamus or pituitary glands, then he's looking at *secondary hypogonadism*. He could also be dealing with *combination hypogonadism,* where he has some level of dysfunction in more than one area.

Think of it like the heating system in your house. You can have problems in the actual furnace (primary) or you can have problems with the thermostat (secondary). Or on some occasions, you may actually have problems with both (combination). Your repairman will tackle each type of repair differently depending on which part is broken.

In the same way, it's important to differentiate between primary and secondary hypogonadism because there are sometimes different treatment options for each. We'll talk about that a little further in this section.

How do you determine whether his low testosterone is primary or secondary? While you can't always know for sure, there are sometimes indicators that can point the way.

Remember that LH (luteinizing hormone) and FSH (follicle stimulating hormone) are produced in the pituitary and are responsible for telling the testes to produce testosterone and sperm. Well, if your husband's LH and FSH values are high but his testosterone is low, for example, it means that his hypothalamus-pituitary glands are doing their job of telling his testes to produce more testosterone, but the testes are taking a little vacation. You know at that point that there's likely a problem in the testes (primary hypogonadism).

If, on the other hand, his LH and FSH values are low even though his T levels are low, then it may be his hypothalamus-pituitary glands that are slacking off (secondary hypogonadism). It's important to note that even if his LH and FSH values are within normal range but his testosterone levels are low, then his LH and FSH levels are 'inappropriately normal' because they actually *should* be elevated in response to his low T levels. This would also tend to indicate that he's dealing with secondary hypogonadism. With combination hypogonadism, LH and FSH levels will vary depending on the circumstances.

## Types of Hypogonadism (Low T)

| | | |
|---|---|---|
| **Primary Hypogonadism** | Problem originates in the testes | LH & FSH levels will normally be elevated while T is low |
| **Secondary Hypogonadism** | Problem originates in the hypothalamus or pituitary | LH & FSH levels will normally be low or inappropriately normal while T is low |
| **Combination Hypogonadism** | Dysfunction exists in both the testes and hypothalamus/pituitary | LH & FSH levels will vary depending on the dysfunction |

Table 4

## Hide 'n Seek with Testosterone

In addition to problems with the hypothalamus-pituitary-gonadal axis, there are problems that can occur further down the line even after a man produces sufficient amounts of testosterone. Many of these issues can be detected through lab work.

It may be that your husband has sufficient amounts of testosterone present in his body, but for various reasons his testosterone may not be usable. As testosterone in the body metabolizes, it can convert into other hormones and into various metabolites, the two primary ones being estrogen (estradiol) and dihydrotestosterone (DHT). As well, the majority of the testosterone a man's body produces is 'bound up' by other substances and isn't usable. Let's look at some of the ways your husband's testosterone may be 'hiding'.

## Estrogen – Too Much of a Good Thing

Many people think of estrogen as a female hormone and are surprised to hear that estrogen also plays a vital role in a man's health. A certain amount of estrogen is important in maintaining a man's heart and bone health, as well as being beneficial to memory and cognitive function. In addition, a certain level of estrogen is needed for a man to have strong erections and libido. However, when it comes to estrogen, a man can have too much of a good thing.

> **Sometimes a man's body converts too much testosterone into estrogen, causing low T symptoms.**

A man's body converts testosterone to estrogen through a process called aromatization. Aromatase is the enzyme widely present in a man's body that converts a small amount of testosterone into estrogen. So far, so good. When the process is working, a man has an ideal testosterone to estrogen ratio and he feels great.

The problem comes in when too much of a man's testosterone is lost to excess aromatase production and he starts converting too much testosterone into estrogen. This can happen for a variety of reasons; including aging, obesity, excessive alcohol consumption, and zinc deficiency, to name a few. It's possible that while your husband's body is producing enough testosterone, he's converting too much of it into estrogen and so the testosterone isn't available to do the work it needs to do.

The other problem with excess estrogen is that there's a feedback loop built into the process so that when a man's body senses that his testosterone or estrogen levels are high, it takes that as a signal to shut down testosterone production. If this is the case for your husband, he may get good results simply from using a med called an aromatase inhibitor (AI) that prevents too much conversion of testosterone into estrogen.

## Total Testosterone vs. Free Testosterone

Testosterone is no good to a man's body if it sits in the testes and doesn't get to the organs and tissues where it's needed. That's why once it's produced by the testicles, it's sent into the bloodstream where it is bound to proteins that help transport it and protect it from being degraded in the bloodstream.

In fact, *most* of a man's testosterone is bound to carrier proteins, leaving only about 2 percent to freely circulate and be used by his body. The unbound, or usable portion is called **free testosterone**.

There are two main proteins that bind to testosterone, **SHBG (sex hormone binding globulin)** and albumin. SHBG binds about 60% of total testosterone in a tight bind that leaves none available to enter cells. SHBG typically increases with age, so as your husband gets older, there is more SHBG to bind his testosterone, leaving less free testosterone available to the tissues and organs that need it. This is why in older men especially, total T levels can be fine, but free testosterone might be deficient.

Albumin binds about 38% of the remaining testosterone in a much weaker bind, allowing testosterone to break free as needed. When you add free testosterone plus testosterone attached to albumin together, you have **bioavailable testosterone**.

Now that you have a baseline of information on how testosterone is made and what can go wrong in the process, we can move on to lifestyle changes that may increase his T levels.

# What to Expect at this Point

- *Now that you know more about what causes low T, you may get a bit fixated on trying to figure out what caused your husband's. Try not to obsess over it because more likely than not you'll never fully know for sure.*

- *You are starting to feel that you're in this together, working together for a common cause.*

- *You're still concerned about whether testosterone treatment is a good option, but you're growing increasingly hopeful.*

# Action Steps

- *Remind your husband that low T is not a death sentence; in fact, it's quite common and easily treatable.*

- *Understand that your husband's best treatment options will be affected by what type of low testosterone he has, whether primary, secondary, or combination, and by what factors are affecting his T levels. We'll be covering this in depth in Stage Three.*

# Chapter 7
# The Holy Grail
## *Lifestyle Changes that Boost T Levels*

A common question for guys who discover that their T levels are low is whether they can boost them through lifestyle changes rather than testosterone replacement therapy. The answer is … sometimes … but not always … and not always by enough.

Obviously, increasing T levels by natural means rather than T therapy is the holy grail, but for many - maybe most - guys, it's simply not possible to increase their levels enough to make a difference. While I've seen some guys have at least some success in this area, I've seen many more who aren't able to raise their levels at all, or are able to raise their levels by only a small amount.

In this chapter, I'll go over some of the lifestyle changes that may increase testosterone levels.

## Will Lifestyle Changes Make A Difference?

It's difficult to know what makes the difference in who will be successful at raising their testosterone through lifestyle changes and who won't. Is it determined by whether the guy has primary hypogonadism versus secondary, or does the type of hypogonadism make no difference at all and there are other factors that we haven't even considered? As you saw in the last chapter, the causes of low T are complex and often murky.

The truth is we simply don't have the hard data to figure it out. Few, if any, definitive studies have delved into this area.

What I *can* say is that the things that raise testosterone levels are also the same things that increase general health and fitness, so it's always a good idea to make the lifestyle changes that might possibly increase T levels in addition to improving physical health. But there are drawbacks to relying *exclusively* on lifestyle changes to correct low T.

## The Downsides

At first glance, there doesn't seem to be a downside to trying to increase T levels through lifestyle changes; however, there *are* actually some hidden pitfalls.

One drawback to relying exclusively on lifestyle changes to increase testosterone levels is that it takes valuable time, and it may be time that your marriage simply doesn't have. By the time a wife in a low T marriage starts looking for answers to her husband's missing libido, the marriage is usually in a dark place. Say your husband takes six months to try natural means of raising his T levels only to find himself no further along than when he started. In that six-

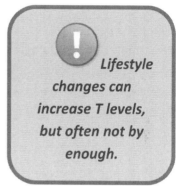

*Lifestyle changes can increase T levels, but often not by enough.*

month period, you will probably see the energy in the relationship decline even further.

Another subtle but important issue with trying natural means is that it typically increases the tension in the marriage. By that, I mean that the wife is usually so motivated for the marriage to improve that she ends up putting a lot of pressure on her husband to keep up all the lifestyle changes.

Every morning he stays in bed instead of going to the gym is a negative for her, and every time she nags him to get up and work out, it's a negative for him. It makes him feel defensive and puts her in the position of being his 'mommy'. Both of these dynamics are disastrous for a marriage that is already struggling in this area.

In addition, most guys with low T levels have a limited amount of energy. The lifestyle changes that raise testosterone take energy … and a whole lot of it! For many guys, it's not realistic to think that they're going to be able to summon the necessary *oomph* to turn things around.

The corollary this is that it's disheartening for a guy to knock himself out making all of these lifestyle changes just to wind up in the same place. I've seen a lot of guys lose heart when their labs show the same low T levels despite months of hard work.

My husband and I experienced this in spades early on in our struggles. He badly wanted to avoid starting testosterone treatment, as did I. For him, it was a matter of being afraid of what T therapy would do to him; for me, it was more that I was very much into a natural approach to life. At that time, I was convinced that a healthy lifestyle was enough to cure any ill that might beset you. I thought that exercise and good nutrition could fix anything. I was wrong.

For a two-year period, he watched his diet like a hawk and worked out consistently while those T levels stubbornly refused to budge. It took a toll on both of us. Every time he got blood work done only to find that his testosterone was the same or even a bit lower, it diminished our hope. Eventually, we became extremely discouraged and almost gave up. In retrospect, we tried the natural approach for far too long.

I find this to be the case for quite a few guys. Here's Ed's experience with trying lifestyle changes:

*"My wife nagged me for years about my life style. My diet wasn't great and I was a couch potato. Once I finally decided to start living healthier, get up off the sofa, and start working out, I expected to see my T levels go up and see some muscle gain. But, nope. Nothing.*

*I intensified my workouts and started eating clean, but still nothing. For two years, neither the weight nor the T levels would budge. And the worst part was that most of it was in my stomach. I didn't know it at the time, but those were my first signs that my testosterone and estrogen were all screwed up.*

*I never expected to have hormone problems. I thought that was for old guys and chicks."*

*--Ed, 46, Industrial Designer*

## A More Measured Approach

What I have found is that it doesn't need to be an either-or approach. In fact, most guys benefit from combining both lifestyle changes *and* testosterone therapy ... at least in the beginning. When your husband starts testosterone therapy at the same time he implements lifestyle changes, there's a fairly predictable progression.

Initially, his energy and motivation are so low that his efforts to maintain his new lifestyle are lackluster. However, as the testosterone therapy kicks in, his energy levels, motivation and mood improve and he starts really rocking the lifestyle changes. He's eager to get to the gym each day, he adds new sports or other activities to his life, and he's more motivated to maintain that healthy diet.

The new lifestyle becomes an integral part of his life and he becomes quite consistent with it. At that point, depending on the original cause of his low T, he may be able to slowly decrease his supplemental testosterone without negatively affecting his T levels. That's how it worked for my husband. Over the last few years, he's decreased his supplemental testosterone several times.

It doesn't work for everyone; for some guys their bodies have simply shut down testosterone production for reasons unknown, and they continue to need that supplemental testosterone. However, it's worth a try. Worst case scenario ... your husband continues to need testosterone, but ends up with much better health and fitness. Best case ... he gets in great shape and reduces the amount of supplemental testosterone he uses.

## Why Didn't It Work?

For those guys who do all the right things - work out faithfully, eat well, get enough sleep, etc. - but see little to no difference in their T levels, their first question quite naturally is "Why didn't it work?"

To which I can only reply, "I don't know." The truth is there's a vast landscape out there that's still murky when it comes to testosterone. We simply don't know all the reasons behind low T.

What we do know is that low T becomes increasingly common as men hit their 30's and 40's. As I mentioned earlier, one large study of almost 1500 men, reported in the *Journal of Clinical Endocrinology and Metabolism,* found that almost one in four men over age 30 has low testosterone levels (defined as under 300ng/dL). Another study showed that 39% of men aged 45 years or older have low testosterone levels.

## TESTOSTERONE DECREASES IN THE LAST TWO DECADES

A study in the *Journal of Clinical Endocrinology and Metabolism* concluded that testosterone levels have declined over the last two decades even after correcting for age, obesity and smoking. This would seem to suggest that something has changed in our current lifestyles and that decreased testosterone levels are not simply a by-product of advancing years.

*"Male serum testosterone levels appear to vary by generation, even after age is taken into account. In 1988, men who were 50 years old had higher serum testosterone concentrations than did comparable 50-year-old men in 1996. This suggests that some factor other than age may be contributing to the observed declines in testosterone over time."*

*Thomas G. Travison, Ph.D., of the New England Research Institutes (NERI) in Watertown, Massachussetts*

What's more, testosterone levels have been dropping in the general population for the last couple of decades. Research shows us that T levels have dropped over the last few decades even after factoring out lifestyle considerations such as age, obesity and smoking.

In other words, a 40-year-old man today with the same general lifestyle as his grandfather has lower testosterone levels than his grandfather did at the same age. That's a startling piece of information!

What's going on with that? Why are testosterone levels dropping in the general population? No one seems to know for sure. There are lots of theories out there ... from estrogen-laden food to pesticide exposure to use of plastics. But at this point, most of it seems to be conjecture. There are small studies here and there that shine some light on the problem, but we lack the long-term, far-reaching, controlled studies that would allow us to draw definitive conclusions.

# Lifestyle Changes that Can Boost T Levels

Okay, while we don't know the whole story as to why testosterone levels decline, we do know at least some things that tend to boost T levels. Keeping in mind that incorporating these lifestyle changes is probably not going to be the holy grail for increasing testosterone, here are some things he can try:

*Get His Beauty Sleep.* It's vital for him to get as close as he can to eight hours of sleep each night. Studies show us that testosterone production drops off quickly and significantly when a man loses sleep. I was amazed at how much impact even short-term sleep deprivation can have on testosterone levels as described in the text box on the next page.

---

*Getting about 20 minutes of bright outdoor light each day and avoiding any electronic light within about 60 minutes of bedtime helps people sleep more deeply and easily.*

---

## INTERESTING STUDY FINDS THAT SKIPPING SLEEP AGES YOUR TESTOSTERONE LEVELS BY 10-15 YEARS

Cutting back on sleep for even a short time drastically reduced testosterone levels in a small group of young healthy men, found a study published in *The Journal of the American Medical Association* (JAMA).

The study took a group of young, healthy men and limited their sleep to five hours per night and then tested their testosterone levels. The testosterone levels were a whopping 10-15 percent lower than when the men got adequate sleep, a decrease equivalent to aging 10 to 15 years!

While this was a very small study, reduced sleep duration and poor quality sleep are known endocrine disruptors, and other studies have also shown a link between lack of sleep and testosterone levels.

One way you can help your husband is to occasionally listen to him breathe while he sleeps. If he snores frequently or stops breathing while he's sleeping, he may have sleep apnea. As I mentioned in Chapter 6, sleep apnea can greatly decrease T levels. It's possible to increase testosterone simply by addressing sleep apnea.

*Lose the excess weight.* Obesity is the condition most commonly associated with low testosterone. Your husband is much more likely to have low T if he's overweight. Of course, it's somewhat of a double bind in that the lower your T levels, the more difficult it becomes to lose weight; so for some guys with low testosterone levels, losing weight is not quite as simple as it sounds.

*Get enough Vitamin D3*. Vitamin D3 is an important precursor to testosterone production. The best way to get Vitamin D is to get out in the sun, but a lot of us can't manage that. The Vitamin D Council recommends roughly 5,000 IU's per day, more if you're deficient. It doesn't matter whether it's liquid, pill or capsule as long as you take it.

*Limit alcohol.* Alcohol takes a toll on testosterone production and one study showed that even moderate amounts for three weeks decreased production by almost 7%.

*Exercise*. While exercise is important to maintaining or increasing testosterone levels, not all exercise is created equal. A body of evidence suggests that HIIT (High Intensity Interval Training) is better at boosting testosterone than other types of exercise. In addition, strength training with higher weights and lower reps, and working large muscle groups seem to be key.

*Manage stress.* If your husband is under chronic stress, his body is producing a lot of cortisol, which blocks production of testosterone. It's impossible to completely eliminate all stress in life, but it's important for him to keep it at manageable levels.

*Lose the Sweet Tooth*. Testosterone levels decrease after consuming sugar. While this isn't a huge problem if your husband indulges only occasionally, if he's eating sugar multiple times a day, he is continually depressing his testosterone production.

*Eat healthy fats*. It's not all about deprivation, however. Another way your husband can increase his testosterone levels is to eat enough fat. That's right; studies have shown that men who have a diet consisting of roughly 20% fat have significantly lower levels of testosterone than men whose diets consist of 40% fat. I'm sure your husband won't mind hearing that particular fact!

Okay, that's it. Those are some things your guy can do to improve his T levels. Nothing flashy, nothing fancy. Just basically doing all the things our mothers told us to do; work hard, eat right, get out in the sun, get lots of sleep, don't drink too much, and have some fun. Doesn't sound all that bad, does it?

# What to Expect at this Point

- *Expect that your husband will want to rely on lifestyle changes exclusively to raise his T levels.*
- *This will probably be frustrating to you as lifestyle changes are slow and their outcome uncertain.*
- *Lifestyle changes take time and energy; your husband will most likely start off strong but he may not be able to last the course.*

# Action Steps

- *Keep making progress through the stages in the book. Go ahead and research doctors, etc. That way, if the lifestyle changes go the way of the dinosaur, you haven't lost too much time.*
- *Let your husband know that while he may implement lifestyle changes, you still want him to talk to a low T specialist in order to get a full understanding of what's involved.*

# Chapter 8
# You Have to Kiss a Lot of Frogs
## *Finding the Right Doc for Low T*

Now that you have a better grasp of the effects testosterone has on your husband and a good feel for where testosterone problems can occur, let's move on to your next step. Do you set up an appointment with your primary care physician? Do you go to one of those walk-in T clinics that have popped up in every strip mall? Do you find a specialist? What's the best approach?

In this chapter, I'll talk about the best ways to find a qualified hormone replacement doctor and the costs of getting T treatment.

Your next step is one of the larger hurdles in repairing a low T marriage. But it's crucial to get it right. While it was fine to use any old clinic to get that initial lab work done, at this point the stakes are much higher. You need to find a doctor who knows what they're doing with testosterone therapy, and I'll give you a clue; unless they have specialized training in this area, it may not be your primary care doctor.

This is the part where I see guys get bogged down and discouraged as they struggle to find someone experienced who's within driving distance *and* takes their insurance *and* actually knows what they're doing. All I can tell you is that you have to kiss a lot of frogs before you find your prince. You may have to switch doctors at least a couple of times before you find someone good.

My own husband went through seven doctors before he found someone with the right kind of training. He saw his primary care doctor first, then a couple of urologists and endocrinologists who didn't have specialized hormone replacement therapy, one holistic doctor who recommended a lot of very expensive supplements, and a guy who specialized in hormone therapy, but who turned out to be too inexperienced to help. We wasted two years and *thousands* of dollars along the way, and I want to help you avoid that.

There's a broad spectrum out there between the drive-thru testosterone therapy clinics where a guy barely has to slow down before they shoot him full of testosterone as he walks in the door, and the holistic doctors who don't want to prescribe testosterone therapy but would rather recommend snake oil and yoga chants. 30,000 *om om om*'s later, your husband's testosterone levels are still tanked.

How do you find someone good?

# Why Can't I Use Just Any Doctor?

The first thing you have to understand is that most doctors get zero training in treating low testosterone while they're in medical school. That's right. Zilch. Zippo. Nada. Bupkas. In his book, *I'm Still Sexy So What's Up with Him?,* Sloan Teeple, MD, mentions how surprised he was when he was diagnosed with low testosterone:

> *"Most surprising of all, perhaps, I had no clue about any of this — and if anyone should have had a clue, it was me. After all, I had studied hard for many long years to become a urologist, a glorified plumber. If any medical doctor should know about testosterone problems, it's a urology resident. But like nearly all of my colleagues, I had received almost no training in diagnosing or treating low testosterone and the life-altering problems that such a condition can provoke."* *(pg. 3)*
>
> **Sloan Teeple, MD**

If a urologist who is trained to study the male reproductive organs gets so little training in testosterone therapy, you can imagine that primary care doctors receive even less.

You'd think you'd have better luck with an endocrinologist. After all, endocrinology is the study of the endocrine glands, the glands that secrete hormones. While there *are* endocrinologists who have extensive training in testosterone therapy, not all of them do. Many men find that the endocrinologist they're seeing focuses primarily on thyroid and diabetes. If you go with an endocrinologist, make sure 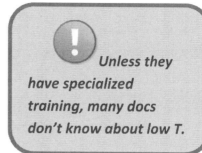 *Unless they have specialized training, many docs don't know about low T.* they've got specialized training in hormone replacement. It's the same thing with urologists. Don't assume they have expertise in this area because of their specialty; check out their credentials specific to hormone deficiencies and therapies before you make an appointment. There's no point in spending money on someone who can't help.

## What about Walk-In Testosterone Clinics?

Your results here would most likely be better than using a doctor with no specialized hormone training at all, but while these clinics are fine for the simple task of getting that initial lab work, they probably aren't your best option for the much more complex job of providing T therapy.

My concern is that many of them have a one-size-fits-all approach. If you're a guy with low testosterone levels, you're probably going to get T therapy regardless of whether other approaches might be a better fit for your situation. In my experience, many of these clinics don't go nearly deep enough to try and figure out the root causes of low testosterone and they typically don't delve into the nutrition and lifestyle issues that affect T levels.

## Who Does This Leave Me With, Then?

Your best chance of finding a doctor who really knows the ins and outs of testosterone therapy is to find someone who focuses specifically on hormone therapy and has specialized training in how to safely administer treatment.

Some of the best doctors I've found have been certified through the A4M (American Academy of Anti-Aging Medicine), or who specialize in

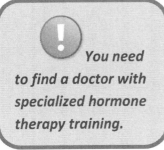

*You need to find a doctor with specialized hormone therapy training.*

'anti-aging' medicine. Additionally, urologists, endocrinologists, and internists who specifically mention hormone therapy on their websites are often good choices. You can google 'anti-aging doctor' or 'testosterone replacement' plus your zip code to find a doctor in your area. Then it's a matter of looking at their website to see what they have to offer.

*Note*: I am not affiliated with the A4M in any way; I have simply seen good results with doctors who are certified through this group.

Once you find a few who look good, check out their websites and if they talk specifically about testosterone therapy, give them a call. Tell the receptionist you're looking for a doctor who specializes in testosterone therapy and ask to speak to someone who can answer some questions for you, preferably the doctor or a nurse practitioner. Table 5 shows helpful questions to ask. Don't be shy about doing this because ruling out doctors who aren't a good fit *before* an initial consultation will save you money in the long run.

## How Much Is This Going to Cost Me?

Many hormone replacement specialists don't accept private insurance. You pay out of pocket and file the bill with your insurance company on your own. They do it this way because they typically spend a lot of time with you, usually between 45 minutes and an hour, and don't want to be constrained to a shorter amount of time by insurance company dictates.

You might be concerned that it will be insanely expensive but that's not necessarily the case. While costs will obviously vary depending on your geographical area, there are ways to keep it affordable. For example, in the Atlanta area, what I've seen is that an initial visit may run between $200-300, with follow-up visits typically being slightly less. Once levels are stable, follow-up visits are usually needed only twice a year. While that's not cheap, you won't have to sell your first-born.

As long as your insurance company will cover your initial and follow-up lab work (and many of them do), then testosterone therapy can be surprisingly affordable even if you're paying out of pocket.

Many of the full service clinics are moving to a concierge system, where you pay a flat fee, which covers a year's worth of care, including lab work and follow-up visits. That's a good model for some people, and allows you to budget for your T therapy at the beginning of the year, knowing what the overall cost is going to be.

> *If your doctor uses a lab that your insurance company doesn't cover, ask about using your own lab. Sometimes a doctor will work with you on this, possibly charging a nominal fee to write orders for the lab of your choice.*
>
> *In addition, some doctors have worked out a deal with a specific lab to get discounted rates on their patients' lab work. Make sure to ask about that.*

## The Biggest Money Saver

I see a lot of guys stumble around when first starting T therapy, trying to utilize their in-network doctors in order to save money. While I'm all for saving money, this is one area where it simply doesn't pay to cut costs. An experienced doctor who can quickly get to the heart of your husband's low T issue will save you money in the long run. A doctor who knows how to look for causes of low T and understands how to effectively administer treatment is worth his weight in gold.

# Questions for Prospective Doctors

Are you a medical doctor? What's your medical specialty? Where did you get your training in testosterone therapy?

How many guys with low T do you see in a typical week? How long have you been prescribing T therapy?

Do you rely only on lab numbers or do you consider symptoms when prescribing T therapy? Is there a specific T level that you aim for?

Do you prescribe HCG and/or Clomid to keep endogenous (internal) testosterone production from shutting down?

What lab work will you initially order? Do you run labs to rule out clotting disorders prior to starting T therapy? Do you run labs before or after the initial consultation?

Do you regularly monitor estrogen levels, hemoglobin/hematocrit levels, and blood pressure?

How do you treat elevated estrogen? How do you treat elevated hemoglobin levels?

Do you perform a physical exam, including a DRE (Digital Rectal Exam)? Do you check bone density prior to starting T therapy?

Do you prefer a specific testosterone delivery mode or do you tailor that to the individual patient?

How often will I need follow-up visits? Are these in-person or via telephone/Skype?

How much will this cost me? Do you have a preferred lab and can I save money by using the lab my insurance company requires?

Table 5

# What to Expect at this Point

- *It's going to be a bit of a rollercoaster as you talk to various doctors. You may get conflicting information. Don't let that throw you, just keep collecting data.*

- *Once you select a doctor, you may feel anxious about the appointment and what the doctor might recommend.*

- *You'll probably experience some concern about finances and whether T therapy will be affordable.*

- *You may feel irritated that you are doing all the heavy lifting instead of your husband stepping up to the plate. Remember he's dealing with a medical issue that affects his energy and focus. It won't always be this way.*

- *You may end up disappointed when you try to discuss all this with your husband and he is less than engaged. This is normal. He's still somewhat in denial and he just wants it all to go away. This attitude will eventually change as you proceed further in the process.*

# Action Steps

- *Research low T doctors in your area.*

- *Call and talk to a few of them directly.*

- *Discuss good prospects with your husband and have him decide which one to use.*

- *Ask your husband to make an appointment that's convenient for both of you.*

- *Call your insurance company to see what your coverage is. Ask them whether there's a certain lab you'll need to use to get the highest level of coverage.*

# Chapter 9
# Human Pincushion
## *First Appointment and Lab Work*

You made it! By this point you've crossed the major hurdles of getting your husband on board and finding an experienced doctor who can help. Congratulations! It took a lot of work and perseverance to get here.

But the new doc you found is requesting a *huge* amount of additional lab work. What's all that about and is it really necessary? Since your husband already got the initial lab work done that showed his testosterone levels were low, you may be wondering what the point is in doing more labs. You've been dealing with this stuff for so long that you'd really just like to move on to a treatment plan.

In this chapter we'll cover what lab work is helpful and how to prepare for that first appointment.

People tend to fall into two camps when it comes to testosterone therapy: those who become paralyzed and do nothing, hoping if they wait long enough the whole thing will go away, and those who want to rush in and solve the problem *now, Now, NOW!* This can be especially true for the wife in a low T marriage, particularly if she's been struggling with the situation for a long time and feels like she's at the end of her rope. Neither approach is particularly good.

While you don't want to sit back and do nothing since low T rarely corrects itself, you can actually do more harm than good by immediately starting T therapy without doing some preliminary lab work first.

Earlier in the book I talked about the many factors that can affect testosterone levels. Now is the time when your husband's doctor will try to identify if any of those factors are at play in your husband's decreased testosterone production.

# Initial Labs

Basically, the more data points your doctor has to work with, the better equipped he is to come up with a treatment plan that works well *for your husband*. Again, low T is not a one-size-fits-all situation. Each man has a different set of risk factors that will determine what treatment plan is best for him. Let's look at some of the labs your husband's doctor will order and why they're being ordered. In addition

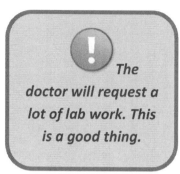

*The doctor will request a lot of lab work. This is a good thing.*

to normal blood work like a lipid panel, a metabolic panel and a CBC, your doctor will probably also want to take a look at the following labs:

**Total Testosterone**: Even though your husband just had that tested, your doctor will most likely want to confirm the results with a second test. Testosterone is delivered to the body in pulses and can vary by as much as 30% over the course of the day, especially in younger men. Your husband's doctor may ask him to get his levels tested as close to 8am as possible since testosterone is highest in the morning, gradually diminishing through the day. He may also have your husband test on an empty stomach since consuming glucose can drop T levels by as much as 25% for as long as two hours.

**Free Testosterone:** The amount of testosterone that's actually available to be used by the body. Because testosterone breaks down into other metabolites and is bound by proteins, free testosterone tells how much testosterone is actually available for his body to use.

**SHBG** (Sex Hormone Binding Globulin): As you may recall, SHBG is a protein that binds testosterone and renders it unusable. If SHBG is elevated, there will be less testosterone available for use where it's needed.

**Estradiol** (Estrogen): You want to establish what your husband's baseline level is prior to starting T therapy for a couple of reasons. If your husband's estrogen is high initially, it might be that by lowering it, his low T symptoms will be alleviated. In addition, testosterone therapy can sometimes elevate estrogen, so it's important to keep an eye on it and make sure it doesn't get too high.

**LH** (Luteinizing Hormone): This is the hormone produced by the pituitary that tells the testicles to produce testosterone. You want to know this level as it provides an important clue as to whether your husband's low testosterone is primary or secondary.

**FSH** (Follicle Stimulating Hormone): This hormone tells the testicles to produce sperm. This is another indicator of whether the low T is primary or secondary.

**TSH** (Thyroid Stimulating Hormone): Thyroid problems quite often go hand in hand with testosterone problems and the symptoms of hypothyroid (low thyroid function) sometimes mimic low T symptoms.

In addition, treating thyroid dysfunction can increase testosterone levels, sometimes making T therapy unnecessary.

**Free T3 and T4:** Additional thyroid measures that give a picture of how the thyroid is performing

**Prolactin:** A hormone produced in the pituitary gland that impacts sex drive, among other things

**Ferritin** (Iron): Elevated ferritin can lower testosterone levels.

**Vitamin D, Zinc & Magnesium**: Deficiencies can lead to lower testosterone levels. Correcting these deficiencies doesn't normally bring testosterone levels all the way up to optimal, but it can help.

**DHEA** (Dehydroepiandrosterone): a hormone produced in the adrenal glands and a precursor to testosterone

**PSA** (Prostate Specific Antigen): Measures a protein produced by the prostate gland. Elevated levels can indicate prostate problems and be a contraindication for testosterone therapy.

## Which Test is Best?

The current gold standard for hormone testing is serum blood levels. While saliva testing and blood spot tests have increasingly become available, there's some controversy as to how accurate they are, with most experts weighing in that saliva testing fluctuates too much to be useful, and that not enough studies have been done to know whether blood spot tests correlate well with clinical symptoms.

The one exception at this time seems to be testing for cortisol, where saliva testing is more accurate than blood levels.

# Summary of Helpful Lab Work

| |
|---|
| Total Testosterone |
| Free Testosterone |
| SHBG - Sex Hormone Binding Globulin |
| Estradiol - Estrogen |
| LH - Luteinizing Hormone |
| FSH - Follicle Stimulating Hormone |
| TSH - Thyroid Stimulating Hormone |
| Free T3 and T4 (additional thyroid measures) |
| Prolactin |
| Ferritin (iron) |
| Vitamin D, Zinc & Magnesium |
| DHEA - Dehydroepiandrosterone |
| PSA – Prostate Specific Antigen |

Table 6

## Prepare for the First Appointment

Your husband has done his part at being a human pincushion, they've taken vials and vials of blood, and his lab results are in. Is it time to see the doctor yet?

Not quite yet. What you'll want to do first is to request a copy of the lab results from the doctor. You and your husband need to get familiar with his labs so you can hit the ground running when you're in the doctor's office. The doctor will cover a lot of ground with you fairly quickly and you don't want to be clueless.

Make two copies of the lab results and bring them to the doctor's office so that both you and your husband can follow along with the doctor as he talks about the labs.

## Bring Written Records

Write down any questions and concerns about the lab work, treatment options, and billing procedures *before* you get to the doctor's office. You're going to be somewhat stressed while you're at the appointment, especially since you're dealing with something as sensitive as low testosterone. It's common to get out of the appointment and immediately remember three really important things you wanted to ask, but forgot.

The doctor will probably ask about any meds or supplements your husband is taking. It helps to have those written down ahead of time. This will allow you to save valuable time during the appointment and will ensure that you don't forget to list something important.

It's also helpful for you and your husband to list all his symptoms as specifically as possible. For example, instead of saying that he's tired a lot,  you should say that he falls asleep in front of the TV four nights each week even though he's getting plenty of sleep at night.

The doctor will probably also talk to your husband about libido and erection problems. Discuss this with your husband prior to going to the doctor's office in order to get on the same page. Remember that it may be tough for him to answer these questions frankly; compassion and understanding on your part will go a long way toward helping him.

Remember that sex frequency chart you did back in *Stage One*? It's a good idea for the two of you to bring that along with you. It's helpful for the doctor to see in writing exactly how much the frequency has declined. You both also need to have a rough idea of how often ED is a problem. The idea is not to make your guy feel bad but rather to give the doctor an accurate picture of what's actually going on. These topics are uncomfortable and being able to hand the doctor a piece of paper with all the information already written down can help it go more smoothly.

The doctor also needs to understand that these issues are having a significant impact on the marriage. These aren't things that need a 'wait and see' approach; rather they need to be addressed as soon as possible in order to repair the marriage. The doctor needs to see the individuals behind the numbers.

## Go With Your Husband to the Appointment

Make sure to go with your husband to his appointment. While this may seem like a strange idea to you, as I've mentioned before, most guys feel extremely uncomfortable talking about low testosterone at first. It's tough for your husband to admit to himself that there's a problem, much less talk about it with a stranger. He'll likely benefit from having your support at his appointment.

Additionally, because the doctor appointment will be stressful for him, it may be difficult for him to focus. By the time he gets home, he may have no idea what the doctor even said. While some doctors are experienced enough to realize this and provide some type of written information, not all of them do and your husband may end up coming home without having gotten the help he needs. After repeatedly experiencing this with my own husband and seeing other couples encounter the same problem, I realized how helpful it is to have an advocate at a doctor's appointment, especially that first one.

## Questions the Doctor May Ask

### Medical History
- How old your husband was when he started puberty and if he had any problems surrounding that
- Whether he experienced any growth issues or ever had a trauma to head or groin
- Whether he had undescended testicles as a baby or whether he's undergone any hernia repair or other genital surgery
- Whether he had the mumps as a child and whether there were any related complications
- Whether he has any chronic diseases or genetic conditions
- Whether he's ever undergone chemotherapy or radiation

### Lifestyle Questions
- Whether your husband is experiencing sleep apnea or other types of sleep disruptions
- Whether he's had an acute illness recently, especially if it required hospitalization or administration of opioid medications
- Whether he has a history of heavy alcohol use
- Whether he's used certain drugs or steroids

### Physical Exam
- Physical exam of the testes to check for varicoceles or other abnormalities.
- General physical appearance, obesity, abdominal fat, and muscle mass
- The doctor may also perform a DRE (Digital Rectal Exam). This is to check for any prostate problems. Along with a PSA (prostate specific antigen) blood test, this helps the doctor rule out prostate problems.

Table 7

In addition, the doctor will be throwing a lot of information your way. While you and your husband are ahead of the curve for having read up on low T, it's still tough to take in all of the information the doctor gives. That's where it's so helpful to take notes. Otherwise, much of what the doctor says will be lost by the time you get home.

You need to be there to provide support and take notes, but try not to take over the conversation. Fill in the gaps as needed, but ideally, you want your husband to develop a good working relationship with his doctor so that he becomes comfortable asking questions and expressing concerns.

## What to Expect at the First Appointment

Your doctor will take your husband's complete medical history and ask a lot of questions. He'll ask general questions about significant stresses and any recent life changes, as well as asking about specific symptoms. Table 7 shows questions the doctor is likely to ask.

## Which Comes First - Appointment or Labs?

In the above scenario, the doctor orders the necessary lab work *before* the first appointment. I've also seen the opposite, where the doctor has the guy come in for the intake appointment, and *then* orders labs based on what was discussed during the appointment. The doctor then does a follow-up appointment, either in person, or via Skype or telephone. Either way works. If your husband has a particular preference, he needs to let the doctor know before the first appointment and see what they can work out.

# What to Expect at this Point

- *There will be a lot of anxiety over what the labs turn up and some confusion as you try to figure out what it all means.*

- *You and your husband may both feel slightly awkward at the idea of you being at the doctor's appointment with him.*
- *You'll feel a huge sense of relief once the doctor's appointment is behind you and you know exactly what you're dealing with.*

# Action Steps

- *Your husband needs to get his lab work done and see the physician.*
- *Obtain two copies of the lab work, one for you and one for your husband.*
- *Go over the lab work with your husband prior to his appointment.*
- *Go to your husband's doctor appointment with him and take notes.*
- *Bring your written notes, including meds and supplements he's taking, sex frequency chart and information about any erection problems.*

# Chapter 10
# The Doctor is In, But Your Husband Is *Not*
## *The Moment of Truth*

Earlier I told you that low T marriages tend to follow a general script. I want to take a quick break here from all the medical stuff and give you a heads-up to prepare you for something I often see at this point.

So far, your momentum has been great. You've made huge progress 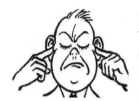 at figuring out the mystery and you've overcome the obstacles to finding a doctor who's experienced enough to help. You and your husband are working together to resolve the issues with your marriage and sex life, maybe for the first time in a long time.

The two of you have found a doctor who looks good and you're ready for your husband to make that initial appointment. You're all excited and tell your husband that this looks like the perfect doc and he should set up an appointment *annnnddddddd* ... he's distinctly underwhelmed. What's going on with that?

In fact, he's telling you that he's decided that he isn't going to make that appointment because there's nothing in the world wrong with him and this is *all in your head*. Quite bluntly, now you're furious. The low testosterone is affecting your whole marriage, you've spent all this time and work to figure out a solution, and he's just going to blow you off?

You hand him this book and tell him to read it. He reads one chapter and tells you that he'll try some natural methods to raise his levels, but that's it. Absolutely no doctors and no T therapy, and he doesn't want to talk about it anymore, thank you very much.

And now you're seeing red. But hold on. Take a deep breath because this is completely *normal*. This is all part of the low T script.

## Giving Up His Man Card

What you have to understand about low T is that it's an incredibly sensitive issue for men. In his mind, if the penis is broke, then he's broke. Most men feel totally emasculated by a low T diagnosis. It makes him feel damaged at a fundamental level, as if someone is asking him to turn in his man card. What he'd really like to do is bury his head in the sand and wait for it to all go away.

What you need to do is defuse the situation as much as possible by reminding him that low T is not uncommon and that it's simply a medical issue that needs to be treated. In the same way that a diabetic needs insulin, a man with low T needs testosterone. Let him know that you'll be with him every step of the way to support him. That you'll go to his doctor appointment with him. That you love him and that the two of you will figure this thing out together.

Stay calm, stay focused. Resist the impulse to give into the anger you're feeling. The day will come when he thanks you for all your hard work and support, but he's not there yet. You have to hold on and be strong for a little while longer.

## Deal Breaker

He needs to understand, though, that this is a deal breaker. This is the point where you have to set a firm boundary. Yes, dealing with the low T makes him uncomfortable, but no more uncomfortable than living in a low-energy, low-sex marriage makes you.

While you may have accepted half of a marriage in the past, you're no longer willing to live with the status quo. Setting firm, loving boundaries is the ticket here.

- *Reiterate to him* that this is a medical issue and medical issues need to be addressed. After all, if your hormones were running amok, your husband would expect you to see a doctor about it and treat the issue. It is *reasonable* for you to want your husband to address this medical issue.

- **Remind him** that this is not just about sex; that it's his health that's at stake and that low testosterone is associated with a number of different health conditions.
- **He also needs to remember** he's not an island. Low T affects his energy and his moods, and that affects the whole family.

# What to Expect at this Point

- *You're both going to be feeling some anger and probably even some grief. This is normal. This feels like a death blow to his manhood and it's a tough time for him. You, on the other hand, are tired of living the way you've been living and you're ready to make some changes.*

- *You may wonder whether addressing his low T is really worth all the angst. There's actually more conflict now than there was before. This destabilization is necessary in order to move your situation forward. It will eventually get better.*

# Action Steps

- *Stay calm and don't give in to the anger you're feeling.*
- *Set boundaries and communicate clearly that this is a deal breaker; you're no longer willing to accept the status quo.*
- *Hold your ground and hang in there.*

# Stage Three

# Fixing the Medical

### The Low T Rollercoaster

*My husband called to give me the 'good news' – his T levels were 234, lower than when he started. We were both devastated. If this doctor, who seemed so knowledgeable and who had been so sure that he knew exactly what to do, couldn't fix things, then who could?*

*This doctor, a urologist, was the fifth we'd seen. Upon his advice, my husband had started applying Androgel every morning. At first, he seemed to have more energy and his libido picked up slightly. Within a month, he actually started feeling good and we felt like we were on the right path at last.*

*However, over the next several weeks, the improvements gradually tapered off and he slipped further back into the low T fog. Our spirits sank. T therapy had been our final option and if it didn't work, then what was left?*

*What had happened? How could his T levels possibly be lower after applying all that external testosterone? The urologist wasn't sure what was going on, but increased the dose, so we crossed our fingers and waited. The Androgel was really expensive, but we were desperate for him to feel better.*

*He again started to see improvements; his energy and libido increased marginally, and at his next follow-up appointment, it turned out that he was at 300ng/dL. His urologist seemed satisfied to leave it there, but we knew this was still far from optimal.*

*We didn't understand why the gel wasn't more effective. At the time, we had no idea that absorption problems are common with topical testosterone, or that he needed HCG to keep his internal production going.*

*We wouldn't learn all that until much later.*

# Chapter 11
# Injections and Patches and Gels! *Oh, My!*
### *Treatment Options Available*

Your husband made it to his doctor appointment. Whew! That's a big step forward. His low testosterone levels were confirmed and based on his levels and his symptoms, the doctor is recommending that he  start testosterone replacement therapy. However, you're both confused about what options are available and which one might be best for your situation. Patches, gels, injections; which is the best option? And what's up with implanting pellets in his hip. That's just plain weird! This whole thing is starting to feel overwhelming.

Don't worry; this chapter will make sense out of all of it for you. There are a number of different options in treating low testosterone, all with different benefits and drawbacks. There's no common consensus amongst doctors as to which testosterone replacement method is best. If you talk to five doctors, you will probably get five different opinions as to the best way to proceed, so let's go over your choices. Table 8 summarizes the various options for testosterone replacement.

I'll also go over some alternative therapies later in the chapter that aren't actually testosterone replacement, but can sometimes boost T levels in certain cases.

***Transdermal methods*** and ***testosterone injections*** are currently the two most commonly used testosterone replacement modes, followed by ***testosterone pellets***, which are quickly gaining popularity. Let's cover those three methods first.

# Testosterone Replacement Products

| Delivery Method | Pros | Cons |
|---|---|---|
| **Transdermals**<br><br>Gels<br>Creams<br>Patches | • Steady, sustained levels<br>• Self-administered | • Possible skin irritation<br>• Frequent dosing<br>• Problems with absorption<br>• Patches are unsightly<br>• Gels & creams can be transferred to others |
| **Injections** | • Cheap<br>• Effective because there's no waste<br>• No risk of transferring to other people | • Peaks & troughs in levels<br>• Semi-frequent dosing |
| **Pellets** | • Steady, sustained levels<br>• Infrequent dosing<br>• No risk of transferring to other people | • Must be administered by doctor<br>• Possible infection at site<br>• Possible extrusion of pellets<br>• Difficult to quickly reverse treatment or adjust dosage<br>• Can be expensive |
| **Buccals/ Sublinguals** | • Steady, sustained dosing<br>• Self-administered | • Possible gum irritation<br>• Visibility<br>• Frequent dosing |

Table 8

# Transdermal Methods

'*Transdermal*' is just a medical term for something that is absorbed through the skin. These types of medications are also referred to as 'topicals' or 'topical meds'. There are a few different transdermal options available; creams, gels and patches. Some are available already prepared and some are individually customized at a compounding pharmacy.

Transdermals are one of the most common methods of testosterone therapy, perhaps because two of the most popular transdermal gels, Androgel and Testim, are still under patent and are marketed heavily to hormone replacement doctors by company reps.

> *Testosterone can either be* Endogenous - *made internally by a man's own body*
>
> *OR*
>
> Exogenous - *added from an external source*

## *Transdermal Creams and Gels*

*Androgel and Testim* are both clear gels and evaporate quickly after being applied due to the high alcohol content. They can be applied to arms, stomach or shoulders, and come in varying dosage levels. Testim has a strong scent, which some people find unattractive. I personally liked the smell of Testim when my husband used it so it's simply a matter of individual taste.

### *Advantages of Gels*
- Deliver a steady, sustained dose of testosterone
- User-friendly without inducing the fear that many people experience with injections
- Easy-to-understand dosing schedule

### Disadvantages of Gels

- Quite expensive unless you have an insurance plan that offers good coverage for them
- Only a small percent of the gel is actually absorbed through the skin into the bloodstream, roughly 10% for most men, with many men absorbing substantially lower amounts. That's simply a lot of waste of an expensive product.
- Another important thing to know is that the gels can be transferred from the user to his wife or children, depending on where he applies it. While most of the gel is absorbed within a few hours, residual amounts may still be present after that.

  Supplemental testosterone is harmful for children, so this is a deal-breaker for some guys. If your husband decides to use a topical, he needs to be sure to wash his hands thoroughly after applying and keep the application site covered to avoid transferring the product to someone else.

Roughly 80-85% of men are able to absorb enough of the creams and gels to see a benefit, and they see results relatively quickly; a couple of weeks for testosterone levels to go up and a month or two for symptoms to improve. If your husband doesn't see a significant increase in his T levels or an improvement in symptoms with the gels within a month or two, he may want to talk to his doctor about either increasing his dose or switching to a different delivery mode altogether.

My own husband got very little benefit from either Testim or Androgel; apparently, he's just one of those guys who can't absorb testosterone through his skin. We sure wasted a lot of money on the gels, and in retrospect, should have switched to injections much sooner. It was discouraging for both of us to spend the time and money on the gels just to see his labs continually come back either no different or actually be lower than when he started. Of course, at the time we didn't know enough to find an experienced hormone replacement specialist; that would have made all the difference.

## Compounded Creams and Gels

These are similar to Androgel and Testim, sharing similar advantages and disadvantages, but instead of being made commercially, they are compounded individually for your husband at a pharmacy. While they are often cheaper and the compounding pharmacy can customize the dosage, quality can be uneven, depending on how good the compounding pharmacy is. In addition, many insurance companies don't offer coverage for compounded meds.

> *A compounding pharmacy is a pharmacy where the pharmacist makes your medication 'from scratch', mixing individual ingredients together based on what your doctor has prescribed.*

## Patches

Like the gels and creams, patches have the advantage of a steady, sustained administration. A man typically applies one or two patches per day, depending on his dosing schedule. Application can be a problem since the instructions state that the patch needs to be applied to an area that is not oily, hairy, nor likely to sweat. They also advise that it be placed in a spot where it will stay flat against the skin and not be pulled, folded or stretched. Now I don't know about your guy, but my husband simply doesn't have many skin areas that meet those conditions! Oh, and he's also advised to choose a different spot each night and wait at least seven days before re-using a spot. Hmmm ... that definitely gets a bit tricky.

In addition to frequent complaints about skin irritation where the patch is applied, another major disadvantage of the patch is that it is on 24 hours a day and thus visible to other people. Some men find this off-putting, particularly in a gym or swimming pool setting. It's simply a visible reminder of an issue that your husband would probably prefer to forget!

### Advantages of patches
- Steady, sustained dosing
- Lower risk of transferring testosterone to other people than with the creams and gels

### Disadvantages of patches
- May be difficult to find a place on skin to adhere to
- Visible 24/7 which is disconcerting for some men

# Injections

Injections are another of the more popular types of testosterone therapy. While many men are initially spooked by the idea of testosterone injections, injections have a number of advantages, the primary advantage being that they are dirt cheap. Testosterone injections have been around since at least the 1940's and thus aren't patented, making them the most cost-effective testosterone treatment for many men.

Some men have their injections done at their doctor's office once every two or three weeks. The disadvantage to this is not only is it inconvenient to have to visit a doctor every few weeks, but your husband will also experience more peaks and valleys in his testosterone levels. To avoid this problem, many men elect to administer their own injections at home, where they can inject as frequently as every three days, keeping their testosterone levels much more stable.

### Advantages of injections
- Cheap
- Cost-effective because there's no waste
- No risk of transferring testosterone to other people

### Disadvantages of injection
- Peaks & troughs in T levels
- Frequent dosing

Now, if you're like me, when I first read that my husband could give himself his own shots, I was a bit freaked out. I mean …. what if he missed the vein? What if he got an air bubble in the needle? What if he got some crazy flesh-eating disease? I pictured my husband grimacing in agony as he bravely injected himself with medication, sacrificing himself for the good of the marriage. All very dramatic, I assure you. I can laugh now at these concerns, but at the time, they seemed very real. I don't like shots, I don't like needles and I don't particularly like doctor visits. This whole thing seemed less than fun!

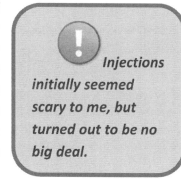

*Injections initially seemed scary to me, but turned out to be no big deal.*

Over time, however, as I did the research, I calmed down. Turns out that testosterone injections aren't administered into a vein at all. Instead, they're **intramuscular (IM)**, meaning that they're administered shallowly into muscle tissue, usually either on his legs or his hip. In addition, the needles are super tiny, very short and thin (or fine-gauged).

My husband currently uses injections, and it's become old hat to us, but this wasn't always the case. When we first started down the road of researching testosterone replacement, somehow I had the idea that it would be this huge, difficult procedure, a major life changer. It did turn out to be a major life changer … in the best way possible! We both had a lot of needless anxiety built up around starting testosterone therapy. Now it's simply a tiny part of our every-day life that pays huge dividends.

For example, the other night we were watching a movie when my husband realized that he had forgotten to inject his testosterone. We paused the movie and in the time it took me to make popcorn, he was done with his shot and we enjoyed our movie together. It's simply not the huge hairy deal that I feared.

## Types of Injectable Testosterone

There are different types of injectable testosterone. Although there is a pure testosterone suspension, it isn't normally prescribed for testosterone replacement because it enters the blood stream too quickly and would have to be administered in small doses several times a day.

Esters slow the release of injectable testosterone from the injection site into the blood stream. An **ester** is simply a carbon chain added to the testosterone molecule that controls how soluble the testosterone is in the blood stream.

Multiple esters can be added to testosterone and each one slows the absorption rate to varying degrees. Some popular ones are:

- ***Testosterone cypionate***
- ***Testosterone propionate***
- ***Testosterone enanthate***

Each type is injected into the legs or hip, where it forms a reservoir of testosterone that gets slowly absorbed into the blood stream. Again, if you talk to five different people, you will probably get five different opinions as to which testosterone ester is the best choice. Your husband will need to find the best ester *for him*.

> *The word 'gauge' (rhymes with cage) refers to how thick a needle is. The higher the gauge, the thinner the needle.*
>
> *For example, a 25 gauge needle is thinner than a 16 gauge needle.*
>
> *Intramuscular testosterone injections are usually administered with a 23 or higher gauge needle.*

For example, my husband did fine on testosterone cypionate for several years. At one point, his doctor wrote a script for testosterone propionate without my husband noticing the change. When he injected the propionate, the injection site became very swollen and sore.

He tried several more times with the same results before giving up and going back to the cypionate. Sometimes it's just a matter of trial and error.

# What's in That Injection, Anyway? Is It Natural?

Your first question when you think about injectable testosterone may be, "What is it made of?" When my husband first started considering T therapy, my gut reaction was fear. For some reason, I pictured him injecting some kind of toxic chemical into his body. I was very much into healthy eating, avoiding modified foods like hydrogenated oils and high fructose corn syrup. The idea of him putting some unknown foreign substance into his body was not a pleasant thought. When your husband uses T injections, what is he actually injecting?

## *Natural vs. Bio-Identical Testosterone*

You often see the phrases 'natural hormones', 'bio-identical hormones', 'synthetic hormones', or 'man-made hormones'. It can get confusing.

Natural testosterone produced in a man's body has a chemical formula of $C_{19}H_{28}O_2$. In order for a testosterone prescription to be *bio-identical*, its chemical structure must exactly match that formula. If you change the testosterone molecule in any way, it is no longer bio-identical.

The various forms of supplemental testosterone are made in labs, mostly from plants like yams and soybeans, so from that standpoint, they can be considered 'natural'. However, they are all chemically synthesized in a lab to get the end product.

So, the only type of absolutely 'natural testosterone' is the testosterone made in a person's body. All other forms are 'synthetic', with some being bio-identical, while others are not.

# Testosterone Pellets

Quickly gaining in popularity, pellets are tiny gel-like objects about the size of a grain of rice that are implanted into the hip and last for four to six months. The insertion needs to be done by a doctor who is qualified, but is an in-office procedure and generally painless. Your husband's doctor will apply local anesthesia and make a tiny incision into the upper hip, placing the pellet inside. There's no need for stitches because the incision is small enough that the doctor usually just closes it with a piece of medical tape.

The benefits of testosterone pellets are that they are absorbed very slowly and don't have the peaks and valleys of injections. Also, once they're implanted, your husband doesn't have to think about them again for months.

Drawbacks are that they can be expensive, the insertion site can become infected, the pellets can extrude out of the skin, and it can be a bit tricky to get the dosing right. However, for some men, pellets are a very good option.

### Advantages of pellets
- Steady, sustained dosing
- Infrequent dosing
- No risk of transferring testosterone to other people

### Disadvantages of pellets
- Must be administered by doctor
- Possible infection at site
- Possible extrusion of pellet
- Difficult to quickly reverse treatment or adjust dosage

## Oral Testosterone

Testosterone should not be taken orally because it is absorbed quickly by the liver where it poses a toxicity risk. If your doctor prescribes oral testosterone, as one of my husband's doctors did, it's an immediate indication that he is not experienced enough to administer your husband's T therapy. Run; don't walk, to a new doctor.

One exception to this is an oral testosterone called testosterone undecanoate that became available in the 1980's. Marketed primarily under the brand name Andriol, testosterone undecanoate works differently than other oral forms of testosterone because it is absorbed into the lymphatic system through the intestines, bypassing the liver.

Because it bypasses the liver, it avoids the liver toxicity problems that beset other oral testosterone products. Not available in the US, one of its chief disadvantages is that it breaks down quickly and thus needs to be administered frequently. The heavy dosing required makes it a pricey alternative to other forms of testosterone replacement.

# Buccal and Sublingual Testosterone

*Buccal treatment* (on the gums) and *sublingual treatment* (under the tongue) are different from oral testosterone because they work by slowly dissolving and being absorbed into the bloodstream without being swallowed, thus avoiding liver toxicity problems. Buccal pellets are usually applied twice a day, once in the morning and once in the evening. For those who don't mind the feel of them, buccal pellets can be a viable option. Sublinguals are usually made by compounding pharmacies, and are typically taken twice a day to get the right dosage. This can make them inconvenient for some men.

### Advantages of buccal/sublingual
- Steady, sustained dosing
- Self-administered

### Disadvantages of buccal/sublingual
- Possible gum irritation
- Visibility
- Frequent dosing

# Alternative & Supplemental Therapies

There are other options that don't actually replace testosterone therapy, but are used either alone or in combination with testosterone replacement to boost internal testosterone production. These options, included in Table 9, utilize different mechanisms for increasing testosterone levels.

## Internal Testosterone Decreases

Once your husband starts undergoing T therapy, the outside (exogenous) source of testosterone will most likely reduce his own internal (endogenous) production by causing his pituitary to stop sending LH (luteinizing hormone) to the testicles.

As I mentioned before, LH is the hormone secreted by the pituitary gland that travels through the bloodstream to tell the testicles to produce more testosterone. The lack of LH from the pituitary causes his testicles to stop producing testosterone. Basically, his testes tell him, "Hey, plenty of testosterone in your bloodstream, we'll take a little break here." Then they kick back and stop doing their job.

This means that initially when he starts T therapy, your husband may experience a surge in his testosterone levels, causing his libido and energy to rise quickly and he'll start feeling great. The problem is that as his endogenous production shuts down, he may actually end up with lower levels than when he started.

Unless he's going to an experienced hormone specialist, his doctor probably isn't going to prepare him for the drop, and both of you will experience a lot of angst once his energy and libido plummet again and you feel like you are right back to where you started. For some men, this can happen very quickly; for others, it can take several months for the endogenous production to shut down. For some men, the drop in endogenous production is severe; for others, it's less noticeable.

## Human Chorionic Gonadotropin (HCG)

This is where **human chorionic gonadotropin (HCG)** comes in. Structurally, HCG is very similar to LH. Because HCG mimics the missing LH and signals the testicles to produce more testosterone, it can help your husband avoid a severe drop in endogenous production when used in conjunction with T therapy.

The combination of increased endogenous production plus exogenous testosterone can help get him to that sweet spot where he's enjoying life again. Anecdotally, many men report an increased sense of libido and well-being when using HCG along with T therapy.

## Options for Increasing Testosterone Levels

**Provides Exogenous (External) Testosterone**

- Transdermal Testosterone
  - Creams
  - Gels
  - Patches
- Injectable Testosterone
- Testosterone Pellets
- Sublingual/Buccal Testosterone

**Alternative/Supplemental Methods that May Boost Endogenous (Internal) Testosterone Production**

- HCG
- Clomid

**Prevents Excess Conversion Into Estrogen**

- Aromatase Inhibitors

Table 9

You may have heard of HCG in connection with the HCG diet. The HCG diet is controversial and has been almost universally discredited as being ineffective and in that context has nothing to do with T therapy.

HCG is a hormone naturally produced in a woman's body during pregnancy. When a woman has difficulty conceiving, HCG is administered to cause ovulation and to treat infertility. It is also used in pubescent boys to correct undescended testes and in men to correct male infertility.

While people sometimes confuse HCG with **HGH (human growth hormones),** they are two very different hormones.

---

*HCG and HGH are two completely separate hormones.*

*HCG stands for Human Chorionic Gonadotropin, and is an important part of testosterone therapy.*

*HGH stands for Human Growth Hormone, and its use is considered controversial by many in the medical community.*

---

## HCG Can Be Used With Testosterone Replacement

Although HCG has been widely prescribed for years for other issues, it is only recently that doctors have started to use it in conjunction with testosterone therapy. Uniform guidelines for HCG administration haven't been developed yet, so you'll find that doctors prescribe varying dosages and frequencies. Doctors who are prescribing HCG to men for fertility enhancement usually prescribe higher doses, while doses for boosting testosterone levels tend to be somewhat lower.

There is some information that suggests that doses higher than 500 IUs of HCG at one time will eventually cause Leydig cell desensitization, thus inducing primary low T where it didn't previously exist. I mentioned earlier in the book that Leydig cells are the cells in the testicles that actually convert cholesterol into testosterone. If they become desensitized, they stop producing testosterone so it's important to make sure the HCG dosage is right.

Your husband's doctor may prescribe HCG to boost endogenous testosterone production at the same time that he prescribes T therapy, or he may wait for a few months to introduce HCG. If the doctor doesn't mention it, your husband needs to bring it up to him to see if it's an option.

One tip I can give you is that because there aren't established HCG protocols, if this is something your husband is interested in, it's imperative to find a good doctor who's experienced in administering HCG to guide him through it. It's definitely not a DIY project.

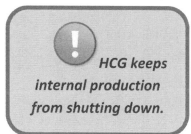

**HCG keeps internal production from shutting down.**

HCG is available commercially or through a compounding pharmacy, and is administered via an injection, much the same as testosterone injections. HCG from compounding pharmacies tends to be cheaper than the commercially available products.

## HCG Can Be Used as Monotherapy

This is a good place to mention a new treatment option that some doctors are using - HCG monotherapy. Monotherapy simply means that HCG is used alone rather than in conjunction with testosterone. I mentioned earlier that low testosterone can be either primary or secondary, originating in either the testes or the hypothalamus-pituitary glands.

Well, if it turns out that your husband's testicles are working fine and his lab work indicates that his low testosterone is secondary (originating in the hypothalamus/pituitary), it's possible that he can increase his testosterone levels by using HCG alone without actually starting on testosterone therapy. The way it works is that once introduced into the bloodstream via self-administered injections, HCG mimics LH, which precipitates the testicles to produce testosterone.

It's important to note, however, that HCG monotherapy won't work for all men. For example, in men whose testicles aren't working anymore (primary hypogonadism), HCG monotherapy isn't the answer. No matter how much HCG you pump in, the testicles simply keep snoozing. However, for those guys whose problem lies in their pituitary or hypothalamus (secondary hypogonadism), HCG monotherapy might be worth a shot.

## Will HCG Monotherapy Work for My Husband?

HCG monotherapy is not nearly as common as testosterone therapy and I'm not aware of any long-term studies that have been done, but at least some doctors have started prescribing HCG monotherapy to their patients. One of those doctors, Eugene Shippen, MD, author of *The Testosterone Syndrome*, has developed a protocol to see whether HCG might be helpful for an individual.

His protocol involves having his patient administer only HCG for roughly a month. At the end of this time period, he measures total testosterone to see if it's increased with the HCG treatment, and based on those results, makes a determination as to whether the man is a good candidate for HCG monotherapy or whether he will need to supplement with traditional testosterone therapy.

Again, while there are no long-term studies on this protocol, it's something you and your husband should know about so he can discuss it with his doctor and determine whether it's something he wants to try.

## Clomid

**Clomid (clomiphene citrate)** is another alternative therapy sometimes prescribed for men who have secondary low testosterone. Clomid is a selective estrogen receptor modulator (SERM), or 'anti-estrogen'. The way it works is that it occupies estrogen receptors, causing the hypothalamus to signal the pituitary to produce more LH. The LH, in turn, travels through the bloodstream to the testicles to spur them into more testosterone production.

Clomid has been used for years in both men and women to increase fertility, and it has a good safety record. Because it was originally approved for increasing a woman's fertility, the doctors who prescribe it for low testosterone do so 'off-label'. There have been some limited studies done recently that show Clomid to be quite effective at boosting testosterone levels without shutting down a man's own internal production. It seems to be especially effective for men in their mid-50's and younger.

## Hey, What Happened to My Testicles?

This may sound funny, but one of my husband's biggest fears about starting T therapy was that his testicles were going to shrink. In fact, when he talked to his GP, the only thing the GP had to say about testosterone therapy was, "Don't do it, it will shrink your testicles." This seemed quite alarming to both of us at the time.

So, *does* testosterone therapy shrink a guy's testicles? Not always, but frequently. Here's the deal. Remember how exogenous testosterone causes a man's pituitary gland to stop sending LH (luteinizing hormone) and FSH (follicle stimulating hormone) to the testes? When that happens, the testicles stop producing as much testosterone and sperm, resulting in testicular atrophy, or shrinking of the testicles.

Because HCG resembles LH, it kick-starts the testicles to once again produce testosterone and helps the testicles return to their normal size.

One of the primary benefits of Clomid is that it not only doesn't hurt a man's fertility the way testosterone therapy can, it actually enhances it. It's not for everyone, but if your husband has secondary low testosterone or if the two of you want more kids, it's worth talking to his doctor about whether Clomid might be a good option for him.

Clomid comes in the form of a small pill and is usually taken several times a week when using it to increase testosterone. Side effects of Clomid are fairly rare and include nausea and vision problems.

What we don't know at this point is whether Clomid is safe for long-term use, so it may be a better option for jump-starting a man's own natural testosterone production or for use only for as long as a man wants to preserve his fertility.

## Aromatase Inhibitor (AI)

I still smile when I think about the time I was talking to a guy about using an aromatase inhibitor, and he thought I was saying he smelled!

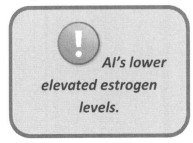

**AI's lower elevated estrogen levels.**

An ***aromatase inhibitor (AI)*** doesn't have anything to do with how your husband smells; rather aromatase is the enzyme in a man's body that converts his testosterone into estrogen, and an AI is a med that prevents that conversion. As I mentioned earlier, while a man needs a certain amount of estrogen in order to be healthy, there are times when his body will convert too much testosterone into estrogen.

A doctor will sometimes prescribe an AI either alone or in combination with T therapy to lower a man's conversion of testosterone into estrogen, thus increasing his testosterone. I've worked with some guys for whom the AI alone was enough to raise their testosterone to a healthy level.

Excess estrogen can cause a man to gain fat, particularly ab fat; it can also cause mood swings and enlarged breasts (gynecomastia). More importantly, high estrogen levels in men are associated with increased cardiovascular problems such as heart attack and stroke.

To monitor estrogen, a lab will test for estradiol, a form of estrogen measured in pg/mL (picograms per milliliter). While most labs use a reference range of less than or equal to 39pg/mL for estradiol, most hormone specialists recommend keeping estradiol lower, somewhere between 20 and 30pg/mL for optimal health. This seems to be the level at which cardiovascular problems are minimized.

While doctors initially prescribed AI's to women who were fighting breast cancer, their use amongst men, especially men using testosterone therapy, has increased in recent years. There are several different types of AI's available, with one of the most common being anastrozole.

Anastrozole comes in the form of an oral tablet, and is available both as a generic and under the brand name Arimidex. Generic anastrozole is very affordable; as an example, my husband uses .5mg three times per week, and pays roughly $6/month.

## You Two Have Some Decisions to Make

Now that you've got a basic idea of the different treatment options, you and your husband have some work to do! You need to decide on the best option for your lifestyle. Does he prefer the pellets so that he doesn't have to think about his testosterone therapy for the next four months or so? Or does the idea of having something implanted in his buttocks freak him out? Is he comfortable with the idea of doing his own injections? Or would he prefer to start off with the transdermals?

These are some of the questions to discuss with the doctor before you decide on a testosterone replacement option. Once the two of you decide on your best option, we can move on to the topic of safely administering testosterone therapy.

# What to Expect at this Point

- *You're likely to feel some anxiety about him starting T therapy, wondering how he will feel and whether it will make a difference.*

- *You may be getting a bit impatient to start seeing improvements.*

- *You'll probably feel somewhat overwhelmed at all the different treatment options. Read up as much as you can and then let your doctor guide you to the best option. Remember, your husband can always switch treatment modes if he needs to.*

- *You'll start to wonder about the safety of testosterone treatment and possible side effects. Don't worry, we're going to cover that in the next chapter.*

# Action Steps

- *Educate yourself about the different treatment options.*
- *Discuss the pros and cons with your husband and get an idea of which treatment method will work best.*
- *Schedule the follow-up doctor's appointment.*

# Chapter 12
# *T Therapy*: The Good, the Bad and the Ugly
## *Keeping It Safe*

Obviously, one of the biggest concerns when a man is considering T therapy is whether it is safe. When we first realized that my husband's testosterone levels were low, we put off getting treatment because we were concerned about the risks.

  To be honest, testosterone therapy simply seemed … *ominous*. Vague thoughts of prostate cancer and shrinking testicles kept us, especially my husband, from wanting to take action. For a long time, we lived in a sort of limbo, kind of hoping that it would all simply go away. But of course, it didn't. In fact, over time as my husband's testosterone levels further decreased, his energy and libido sank even lower.

Low testosterone rarely fixes itself. Your husband is not going to wake up one morning 'cured' of his low testosterone. In fact, without intervention, after the mid-30's testosterone levels mostly go in one direction … *south*. Sooner or later, your husband is going to have to address the problem despite his fears. As it turned out for my husband and me, most of our concerns had no basis in fact and the things we *should* have been concerned with weren't even on our radar!

Remember that in starting T therapy, your husband is simply adding back something his body already makes. Unlike other medications where you introduce a foreign substance into the body, your husband will simply be supplementing his own body's normal production of testosterone, bringing those levels back to where they used to be.

However, that being said, there are some conditions that contraindicate T therapy and there are also some conditions that can arise as a result of T therapy. First, I'll go over some common concerns about testosterone therapy, and then later in the chapter I'll cover conditions that preclude its use. After that, we'll talk about problems that can arise from using T therapy and how to detect and treat them.

# Is He Going to Get Prostate Cancer?

Let's tackle the biggest fear first. Prostate cancer. This is a huge fear for a lot of guys. People are terrified of prostate cancer, and rightfully so. Prostate cancer is the most common cancer amongst men and the second most common cause of cancer death. Given these stats, it's obviously crucial to know whether testosterone therapy increases your man's risk for prostate cancer.

## *What Is the Prostate?*

First of all, what is the prostate? If you're like I was, you may be a bit cloudy on what the prostate even is. The prostate is a gland a little larger than a walnut located on a man between the bladder and the penis. It produces a fluid that makes up semen and it's also responsible for expelling semen during ejaculation.

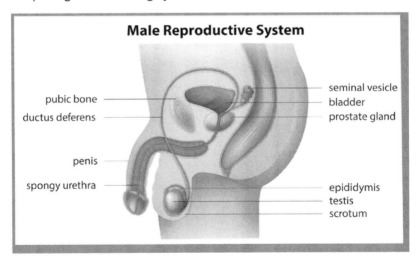

**Male Reproductive System**

pubic bone
ductus deferens

penis
spongy urethra

seminal vesicle
bladder
prostate gland

epididymis
testis
scrotum

## *The Rumors*

For a long time, there was a general belief in the medical world that high levels of testosterone increased a man's risk of prostate cancer. Given this belief, what does the research actually tell us?

## The Research

The truth is that testosterone therapy doesn't cause prostate cancer; in fact, it doesn't even increase a man's risk. Study after study has borne this out, with one of the most important being a study published in the *Journal of the National Cancer Institute*. The researchers took data from 18 separate studies and looked at the relationship between testosterone levels and prostate cancer. Here's what they concluded:

*"(Original data was collected from) 18 studies and analyzed … to determine the relationship between blood levels of sex hormones and prostate cancer. The pooled data included 3,886 men with prostate cancer and 6,438 controls.*

*The researchers found no association between prostate cancer risk and blood levels of different forms of testosterone."*

If this is the case, then why do concerns about testosterone and prostate cancer persist in people's minds?

Well, in men who already have prostate cancer, an effective form of treatment is lowering their testosterone to castration levels. In fact, at one time castration itself, which eliminates the body's supply of testosterone, was a first-line treatment for prostate cancer. A harsh solution, to be sure, but an effective one.

In the 1980's, a new treatment involving a medication that lowered testosterone levels was developed, drastically reducing the need for castration. But here's the catch … testosterone levels need to be close to castration levels, more specifically, under 50ng/dL in order to effectively prevent the recurrence of prostate cancer.

In other words, once you exceed this very low castration level of testosterone in the body, the prostate becomes 'saturated' with testosterone and adding more doesn't change the concentration of testosterone in the prostate at all. Think of it like a measuring cup. Once you fill it to the brim, the rest of the fluid simply pours over the sides.

Once it's full, it doesn't matter how much more you add, it can't get 'fuller'. With prostate cancer, once you exceed the 'saturation level' of the prostate, adding more testosterone simply doesn't matter.

> **Research shows us that T therapy doesn't cause prostate cancer.**

So in men whose testosterone levels have been medically lowered as part of their treatment for pre-existing prostate cancer, it's possible that changing their testosterone levels can cause already occurring cancer cells to regrow, but in men who don't have pre-existing prostate cancer, testosterone therapy doesn't raise their risk.

Abraham Morgentaler, MD, author of the book, *Testosterone for Life*, gives a fascinating account of the twisted tale of the misconceptions about testosterone and prostate cancer. It's well worth the read if you'd like the full story. After years of studying the topic, here's what he has to say:

> *"In 2004, when my article in the* **New England Journal of Medicine** *was published, there were fifteen of these longitudinal studies examining the relationship of hormones and prostate cancer. Since 2004, there have been approximately a half-dozen more. Not one has shown any direct relationship between the level of total testosterone in a man's blood and the subsequent likelihood that he will develop prostate cancer. Specifically, average total testosterone levels were not higher in the cancer group compared to men without cancer, and men with the highest T values were at no greater risk for later developing prostate cancer than men with the lowest T values."*

> "Destroying the Myth About Testosterone Replacement and Prostate Cancer."
> *Life Extension Magazine* Dec 2008: Web.

Furthermore, not only is there no correlation between high testosterone levels and prostate cancer, there's actually information that suggests the opposite ... that men with **lower** testosterone levels have a greater risk for prostate cancer.

Multiple studies have confirmed this. One such study of 206 men reported in the *World Journal of Urology* states that, "This study supports experimental findings that testosterone levels are predictor of prostate cancer and that prostate cancer is frequently associated with **low testosterone levels**." (Emphasis mine.)

In another study of 568 men, the conclusion drawn was that, "Patients with lower levels of serum testosterone had a higher risk of prostate cancer than did patients with high serum (blood levels of) testosterone."

---

*The word 'prostate' has only one 'R' in it.*

*It comes from the Greek 'prostates'; meaning 'to stand before, because the prostate 'stands before' the testes.*

*Not to be confused with the word 'prostrate', which means to lie flat.*

---

## Tests to Rule Out Pre-Existing Prostate Cancer

Now that you have an understanding of the relationship between testosterone and prostate cancer, you can see how important it is to rule out prostate cancer prior to starting on testosterone therapy. How do you do this? An experienced doctor will administer two tests to rule out existing prostate cancer before he recommends T therapy:

- **DRE (Digital Rectal Exam)**
- **PSA (Prostate Specific Antigen)**

Most guys like having a DRE performed about as well as most women like getting their annual Pap smear; however, performing a DRE allows your husband's doctor to manually feel for enlargement, lumps, or irregularities that are indicators for prostate problems.

The PSA is a simple blood test that also helps detect problems with the prostate. Taken together, the two tests provide a good screening mechanism prior to starting T therapy. As long as the two tests are normal, testosterone therapy can be considered.

# Is He Going to Have a Heart Attack?

Another concern I had when my husband was considering testosterone therapy was whether he would be at higher risk for a heart attack, a reasonable concern given that the number one killer of Americans is heart disease.

## *The Rumors*

At one time, there was a belief in the medical community that the higher testosterone levels in men were responsible for the higher number of heart attacks and strokes that men had compared to women with their lower testosterone levels. However, research indicates that not only is this not the case, it seems that *lower* testosterone levels are actually a risk factor for heart disease.

## *The Research*

One large study followed 2,416 men for five years. Men with higher testosterone levels had a 30% lower risk of having cardiovascular events (heart attacks, strokes, etc.). Men with the lowest testosterone levels were twice as likely to have cardiovascular disease. Multiple studies bear out similar findings.

The data is not as clear for men who are older than 65 and in poor health. Some recent studies have suggested that testosterone therapy in this population can increase risk factors. However, the studies didn't control for important variables like estrogen levels and hematocrit levels, which in and of themselves can be risk factors for heart events. This limits the usefulness of the studies when making a decision about testosterone therapy in men over 65.

# Is He Stuck Doing T Therapy Forever?

This is a common concern for many men. There's this thought that once they start on T therapy, it's an irrevocable decision and they can't ever stop. A fairly chilling thought.

This is not the case, though. Your husband can stop testosterone therapy any time he wants. Now the catch to that, of course, is that he'll stop feeling the benefits of the higher testosterone levels and he'll go back to experiencing the usual low T effects of fatigue, loss of libido, lack of focus, less positive moods, etc.

In addition, if he wasn't taking HCG to keep his own internal production going, he could end up worse off than before because the testosterone therapy will have shut down his own production. However, for some men, it's possible to restart his own internal production with HCG monotherapy. While testosterone treatment is not a decision to be made lightly, it's also not a permanent, irrevocable step that can't ever be changed.

# Will He Turn into a Raging Maniac?

Another very common fear for men is that if they start taking testosterone, they will turn into raging maniacs. Maybe it's something you're worried about as well. The reality is that 'roid rage is typically confined to those men who take excessively high doses of various steroids in order to achieve supra-physical levels of performance.

Most guys who are simply replacing their testosterone levels to get back to where they were when they felt their best are not going to turn into aggressive jerks. In fact, the opposite is true. Many men feel tense and irritable when their testosterone levels are *low*.

For the vast majority of men, raising their testosterone to optimal levels typically helps them become more cheerful and stable. They are calmer, they sleep better, they feel a sense of well-being, and they regain their zest for life. This was very much the case for my husband; it's like I got back the guy I married - the one who had disappeared for so many years!

# Contraindications for T Therapy

There are conditions which make T therapy a poor choice for some men. These include clotting disorders, pre-existing prostate or breast cancer, and untreated sleep apnea. I've already talked about prostate cancer, but let's go over complications caused by clotting disorders and sleep apnea.

## *Clotting Disorders*

There is a small group of men who have rare blood-clotting disorders who should not take testosterone therapy. These clotting disorders interact with testosterone therapy to produce dangerous and even fatal blood clots. They are so rare that many books and articles about testosterone therapy don't even mention them, but because they can be so dangerous, it's important for you to know about them.

Fortunately, there are simple blood tests to rule out these types of clotting disorders, available with your other blood work at your regular lab and routinely covered by health insurance. Charles Glueck, MD, of Jewish Hospital Cholesterol and Metabolism Center, recommends testing for blood clotting disorders prior to starting testosterone therapy, including tests for Factor V Leiden, Prothrombin gene, Factor VIII and Factor XI. It's important to do these tests because many people with clotting disorders are asymptomatic and have no idea that they have one.

## *Sleep Apnea as a Risk Factor*

Let's talk about snoring. Not all that glamourous, I know, but it turns out that severe snoring can sometimes be a sign of sleep apnea. Sleep 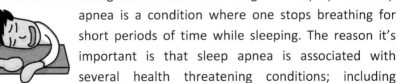 apnea is a condition where one stops breathing for short periods of time while sleeping. The reason it's important is that sleep apnea is associated with several health threatening conditions; including obesity, cardiovascular disease and high blood pressure, diabetes, anxiety, and depression.

Sleep apnea also has implications for testosterone therapy. The relationship between testosterone and sleep apnea is tricky. On one hand, men who have sleep apnea tend to have lower testosterone levels. On the other hand, at least in one small study, when men with sleep apnea started testosterone therapy, the sleep apnea got worse.

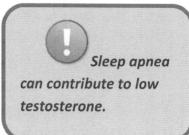

*Sleep apnea can contribute to low testosterone.*

What does this mean for you and your husband? If he is a heavy snorer, or if you notice that he sometimes stops breathing for short periods while he sleeps, he needs to get in for a sleep study. While many guys dislike the inconvenience of a sleep study, it's important because of the impact that sleep apnea has on his overall health, energy, and libido levels. In addition, many hormone replacement specialists will not prescribe testosterone therapy to a man with untreated sleep apnea.

My husband snored for years and frequently stopped breathing at night. His snoring and snorting would keep me awake to the point where I felt like kicking him! But I would also anxiously listen for him to start breathing again. Given the fact that he snored so heavily for so many years, it's not surprising that he ended up with low T. Although we didn't know it at the time, testosterone and sleep apnea go hand in hand.

When we finally realized that he was at risk for sleep apnea, the whole idea of getting a sleep study seemed overwhelming to us. We weren't sure where to start in terms of seeing our general practitioner or a specialist. We also weren't sure how much it would cost and how much insurance would cover. The whole thing sounded inconvenient and time-consuming.

## Treating Sleep Apnea

However, it turned out that it wasn't that big of a deal. If you and your husband are dealing with this, he can go to his family doctor and let him know that he suspects sleep apnea. The doctor will either write a script for a sleep study himself, or refer your husband to a specialist who will actually order the sleep study. If the sleep study shows that he has sleep apnea, the doctor will probably prescribe a **continuous positive airway pressure machine (CPAP)**. These are small machines that have a mask that fits over the nose and/or mouth and provide continuous pressure in order to keep the airway open.

It takes a while to adjust to a CPAP machine because it can be irritating to have to wear a mask to bed. However, the benefits of waking up feeling rested and being able to stay alert during the day usually win him over fairly quickly.

I have seen men benefit from treating their sleep apnea almost as much as they did from starting testosterone therapy. They simply feel so much better that the inconvenience of the CPAP machine is well worth it.

My own husband hated the idea of getting a CPAP because he didn't like the idea of being tied to a machine at night. However, once he started using it consistently, he felt so much better during the day that he was sold. No more falling asleep during meetings, no more falling asleep on the sofa at night.

He did have to play around a bit to find a mask that was comfortable. There are multiple types and some work better than others. I'm a light sleeper, and I was concerned that sleeping next to him while he used a CPAP would be like sleeping in an airport terminal, but the machine is actually fairly quiet. There is a faint hum, but nothing that's detectable over the whir of our overhead fan.

Oral devices are a fairly new option out there for sleep apnea. According to the *American Sleep Apnea Association,* there are over 80 different oral device models available for treating mild to moderate sleep apnea. While I don't have any personal experience with them, I've heard guys say that they had good results using the oral devices. If your husband's sleep apnea isn't severe, it might be worth asking the doctor about an oral device rather than a CPAP machine.

Most insurance companies cover both the cost of the sleep study and the CPAP machine, so getting this condition taken care of is mostly painless. You just have to get past the dread of making those initial phone calls to the doctor and insurance company. I think you'll find that the benefits make the effort well worth it.

# Conditions that May Result from T Therapy

As I mentioned in the beginning of the chapter, there are some conditions that can affect health as a result of using T therapy. It's important that your husband's doctor monitor them.

## *Elevated Hematocrit*

Testosterone stimulates red blood cell production. This can be a great thing for those guys who are anemic (not enough red blood cells); in fact, at one time, testosterone treatment was prescribed to treat anemia. However, for a man who already has healthy red blood cell levels, testosterone therapy can cause his red blood cell levels to increase too much, a condition 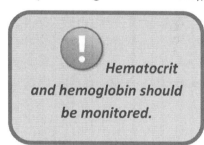 called **erythocytosis**, or **polycythemia**. This can cause his blood to become too thick, making it tougher for his heart to pump it, which can contribute to cardiovascular issues.

*Hematocrit and hemoglobin should be monitored.*

Testosterone therapy usually raises **hematocrit** (the part of the blood composed of red blood cells), typically by about three percent. An experienced hormone replacement specialist will regularly monitor your husband's hematocrit to make sure it stays at a healthy level. Some doctors also monitor **hemoglobin** (the part of the blood that transports oxygen and gives blood its red color).

Different doctors have different guidelines about how often to test these levels, but at a minimum, they need to be checked prior to starting testosterone therapy and then within three to six months after starting treatment, and once or twice a year after that.

My husband, for example, gets his checked anytime he goes to his hormone specialist and gets blood work done, usually two to three times per year.

## How to Handle Elevated Hematocrit

If the hematocrit gets too high, there are several different options to correct it. Your husband can always lower his dosage, or even discontinue T therapy altogether. If he is using injections, he can try switching to patches or gels as these treatment modes seem to be less likely to raise hematocrit than injections.

However, your husband may be reluctant to give up the benefits of testosterone therapy once he starts. For a lot of guys, periodically donating blood is enough to sufficiently lower the hematocrit count. Typically, once every two or three months is enough to resolve the problem, depending on how high his hematocrit is.

It's a good idea to keep a log of hematocrit and possibly hemoglobin levels, along with the date when he last donated blood. This lets him stay on top of his blood donations and make sure they happen as often as needed.

## Elevated Blood Pressure

In rare cases, testosterone therapy can raise a man's blood pressure. Thought to be caused by water retention and the increase in red blood cells, increased blood pressure occurs more often in men who are using excessively high dosages. However, even for guys who are only on replacement doses, it's still a good idea to get blood pressure readings prior to starting testosterone therapy and periodically after that.

## Dangers of Elevated Estrogen

As I mentioned earlier, elevated estrogen has been implicated as contributing to both heart attacks and strokes, so your husband's doctor will monitor his estrogen with the goal of keeping it somewhere between 20-30 pg/mL.

Estrogen should be tested prior to a man starting testosterone therapy, and again a few months after he begins T therapy. Thereafter, it should be tested at least once or twice a year.

## *Gynecomastia aka 'MOOBS'*

When I first heard the word 'moobs', short for man-boobs, I had to laugh. While the word sounds pretty silly, gynecomastia (enlargement of a man's breasts) isn't funny to the guy who's experiencing it. Gynecomastia can sometimes be accompanied by tenderness or itching of the nipples and is usually caused by elevated levels of estrogen, another important reason for your husband's doctor to monitor his estrogen levels. Once the estrogen is lowered via an aromatase inhibitor, the gynecomastia usually disappears.

## *Low Sperm Count*

Testosterone therapy normally lowers sperm count, something that doctors don't always remember to tell a patient. As I mentioned earlier, once there is testosterone in a man's blood stream, it causes his pituitary gland to stop sending LH (luteinizing hormone) and FSH (follicle stimulating hormone) to the testes. When that happens, the testicles stop producing testosterone and sperm.

> **T therapy usually reduces sperm count unless you add HCG.**

If you and your husband want to have (more) children, your doctor will most likely recommend against traditional testosterone therapy. He may instead recommend Clomid (clomiphene citrate) or HCG to raise your husband's endogenous production of testosterone while preserving or even enhancing his fertility.

If your husband has already started on testosterone therapy and the two of you still want kids, don't panic. Low sperm count is normally temporary and typically resolves once a guy discontinues testosterone therapy. Some guys are back to normal within a month or two, while for others it takes considerably longer. In those cases, it may be worth taking a look at Clomid or HCG to spur sperm production.

## Conversion to DHT

The body converts some testosterone into DHT (dihydrotestosterone). While DHT typically increases libido, in excess amounts it can cause acne, hair loss and possibly prostate inflammation. Your husband needs to monitor his DHT in order to keep it within optimal range.

## Acne

Testosterone treatment sometimes causes acne because it stimulates the sebaceous glands and they produce excess oil. For most men, the effects are usually fairly mild and seem to subside after several months of treatment. At least some studies show that supplementing with anywhere between 200-600mg of zinc daily can improve acne. Since correcting a zinc deficiency can also increase testosterone production, this would seem to be a win-win.

## Hair Loss

One concern my husband had about starting T therapy was that it would cause him to lose his hair. Although there are anecdotal reports that testosterone therapy accelerates balding, there are no reliable studies that have been done on the topic. Hair loss seems to be primarily determined by genetics, and the jury is still out as to whether testosterone therapy influences that.

I've read accounts of men who have used finasteride (common brand name, Propecia) to slow hair loss. Finasteride works by inhibiting the conversion of testosterone into dihydrotestosterone (DHT). The problem with this is that reducing DHT can also reduce libido, erections, and sperm volume, at least for some men. What's more, for some men the results seem to be permanent. My advice here would be to tread carefully with the use of finasteride and be aware of potential side effects.

# Additional Lab Work

There are a few other labs that are helpful for your doctor to order before your husband initially starts T therapy and then periodically after that.

## Bone Density

It's a good idea for your husband to ask his doctor to check his bone density before starting testosterone treatment. Not because T therapy hurts bone density, but because low testosterone is associated with osteoporosis. Testing bone density will show whether there's a problem that needs to be addressed. A bone density test takes about five minutes utilizing a machine that uses a tiny amount of radiation, much less than a standard X-ray.

If the test is normal, it doesn't need to be repeated for a few years. If the test shows that bone density is compromised, your husband will need to discuss treatment options with his doctor. Sometimes, testosterone therapy alone will bring bone density back into normal ranges, depending on how severe the bone loss is.

This test isn't absolutely necessary, but if your insurance company will cover it, it's good information to have.

## Testosterone Levels

This may seem obvious, but it's important to actually monitor testosterone levels after starting T therapy. Your husband will need to know what his levels are prior to starting therapy, and then again at roughly four weeks after starting. When your husband hits the sweet spot where he's feeling wonderful, it's a good idea for him to get a blood test drawn to find out where his levels are so that he knows what he's aiming for. Thereafter, it's normally necessary to monitor levels only twice per year.

If your husband is using injections, he needs to get his blood work done just prior to his next injection. Most doctors will try to keep testosterone levels between 500 and 900 ng/dL. My experience is that most men need to be at 500 ng/dL or above in order to feel fully sexual;

some of them need to be well over 500. My own husband seems to do best somewhere between 700 and 800 ng/dL. Each man will have to experiment a bit to find his best level.

Because the ideal testosterone level is individual to each man and the doctor will rely on your husband's subjective report when determining the best testosterone dose, it's vital that your husband is honest with his doctor about how he's feeling. This is no time for a stiff upper lip. He needs to let his doctor know how his energy and libido are doing, whether he's still experiencing ED, whether he's sleeping well, etc.

One tool I've found helpful is to ask a man to describe his energy and libido on a scale of 1-10. Asking him to quantify it in this way allows him to accurately report how he's doing without him feeling like he's complaining. Go ahead and log these numbers on a weekly basis along with his most recent testosterone and estrogen levels. This will give you a feel for where his sweet spot is. You can keep all this information together along with lab results, office reports, and dates of blood donations.

It's important to note here that his T levels will take a while to stabilize. You're going to see some peaks and valleys for a while. The doctor will probably have to tweak his doses for testosterone, HCG and the AI for a bit before it levels out. More experienced doctors are normally able to get him to that sweet spot quicker.

# Labs Needed to Safely Monitor T Therapy

Now that you understand some of the conditions that can contra-indicate T therapy, as well as some conditions that can result from it, you can see how important it is for your husband's doctor to run labs that monitor the conditions.

Table 10 summarizes the specific labs and tests your husband will need along with his normal blood work in order to safely begin and continue with testosterone replacement.

# Important Tests for Safely Administering T Therapy

| |
|---|
| Hematocrit and Hemoglobin Levels |
| Blood Pressure |
| Estrogen (measured as estradiol) |
| PSA and DRE (prostate) |
| Total and Free Testosterone |
| Tests for Blood Clotting Disorders (prior to starting testosterone treatment) |
| Bone Density Test (optional but helpful) |

Table 10

## Your Role is Vital to Keeping T Therapy Safe

I've gone over a lot of medical jargon with you in this chapter, but let me take a minute to bring it back to the personal level. I know that this is all a lot to take in and you may be feeling overwhelmed at this point by all you need to know. You may simply be tired of dealing with all his medical stuff. You're ready to hand it off to him and let him do his own monitoring, tracking and ordering.

I urge you to hold off for a bit longer. It's going to take a while for that low T fog to clear away enough that he's capable of taking hold of the tiller. It will come, but not quite yet. You'll do yourself a tremendous favor by keeping tabs on all this until he's able to steer his own ship.

For now, you need to stay on top of the action steps until he's ready to take over; your participation is vital in helping the transition go smoothly and making sure that nothing falls through the cracks.

## The #1 Safety Factor for T Therapy

In conclusion, like any other medical treatment, testosterone therapy has risks and benefits. It is safe when administered correctly, but in the hands of an inexperienced doctor, there can be risks. Make sure your husband has a doctor who understands the importance of checking for known risk factors and contra-indicators for testosterone therapy. You want someone who looks at your husband as a whole person, rather than a lab number.

Testosterone therapy is not a one-size-fits-all situation and an experienced doctor will request a battery of tests in order to determine particular risk factors for your husband and the best way to treat his specific situation. Finding an experienced doctor who knows how to safely and effectively administer T therapy will save you time and money in the long run. More importantly, you'll both have peace of mind.

# What to Expect at this Point

- *His T levels will be up and down for a while as the doctor adjusts his dosage. These will stabilize over time.*

- *Your interactions are probably getting more productive at this point. There's less anxiety and anger as the two of you adjust to the new normal.*

- *As his T levels stabilize, you're both starting to feel much more settled and hopeful that your marriage will start changing for the better.*

- *You may feel impatient to see results. You need to be patient here; this is a process.*

# Action Steps

- *Rule out sleep apnea and if it seems to be a problem, set up a sleep study.*
- *Keep track of testosterone levels and the effect they have on how your husband feels.*
- *Keep track of his hematocrit levels. If he donates blood, keep track of when.*
- *Keep track of estrogen so that it doesn't get too high.*
- *Keep tabs on his meds and when to re-order.*

# Chapter 13
# It Sounds Too Good to Be True
## *Benefits of Testosterone Therapy*

Yay! Your husband started his T therapy! It's been a long journey to get to this point. My husband and I travelled the same long path and I know how difficult it's been. Congratulations on your hard work and your perseverance.

Now comes the moment of truth where you find out whether all of your hard work is going to pay off. You may be wondering if testosterone therapy is too good to be true. Will it really help your husband feel better and benefit your marriage?

In this chapter, I'll go over what you can expect to see in the next few weeks and months now that your husband has started testosterone treatment.

While testosterone therapy is not a magic bullet, the truth is that **hormones matter**. Eugene Shippen, MD, author of *The Testosterone Syndrome*, sums it up this way:

> *"I have measured the testosterone levels of many hundreds of men, and I have never seen an older male in excellent mental and physical health whose testosterone levels were not well within the normal range. And the healthiest, most vital individuals are always in the high normal ranges." (p. 5)*

## How Long Before You See Results?

The first question for a guy who has started T therapy (and his wife!) is always, "How long does it take to see results?"

This varies widely. Some men see results almost immediately; for others it can take a few weeks to a few months. He may see quicker results in his energy levels and mood than he does in his sex drive. It really depends on the guy.

## Libido

Let's be honest, a dwindling sex life is what started most of us on the search for a solution. If you're like many women, the crucial question is whether testosterone treatment will fix his sex drive. Or at least improve it.

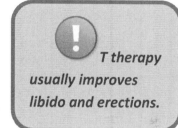
*T therapy usually improves libido and erections.*

For most men, the answer is yes. One of the primary symptoms of low T is a lowered sex drive. Assuming that your husband's sex drive was normal when he was younger and had higher testosterone levels, and assuming that his sex drive is not getting siphoned off into porn or another woman, then it is very likely that you are going to see an increase in his libido once he starts T treatment.

Will your husband be the crazed sex maniac that you would like him to be? Well, maybe not right away. There's often some healing that has to take place, especially if his confidence has been shot either by the low T itself or from bouts of ED. While testosterone fuels libido to a certain extent, sexuality is complicated. Confidence drives a man's desire to initiate sex. Your husband has been through a difficult medical issue; it will probably take him a while to recover enough to become that confident lover he used to be.

However, healthy testosterone levels form the foundation for the healing to take place. One large study of 1632 men reported in *The Journal of Clinical Endocrinology and Metabolism (JCEM)*, concluded that "libido and T concentrations are strongly related" and that "T supplementation has been associated with increases in sexual functioning, mood, and strength."

## Better Erections

I want to cover an area where people tend to get confused. Libido and erectile function, while related, are two separate issues. Libido refers to a man's *desire* for sex; erectile function has to do with his *ability* to have sex. **Erectile dysfunction** is defined as the inability to get or maintain an erection.

Leaving libido aside for the moment, let's talk about erectile dysfunction on its own. Low testosterone and ED don't perfectly correlate; that is, some men with low T are still able to get great erections while others suffer from ED even when their T levels are high. Your husband may never have had a problem with erections even when his testosterone was at his lowest. Another guy may continue to struggle to have strong erections even after he starts T therapy.

However, that being said, even though the two aren't *perfectly* aligned, low T does usually have an impact on erectile function, and for many men, fixing the low T can have a significant impact on their ED.

In one study of 211 men, roughly 60 percent of them saw improvement in their ED after they started T treatment. In addition, for men who didn't get good results from using Viagra alone, testosterone therapy in combination with Viagra increased their rate of success.

Multiple factors affect erectile function; high blood pressure, circulation issues, diabetes, stress, fatigue, injury to the penis, smoking, alcohol consumption, and certain medications. While testosterone treatment is a good starting point, sometimes it's not enough. We'll cover other treatment options for ED in greater detail later in the book.

## Increased Energy and a Zest for Life

While my husband's lack of sex drive was the number one thing that drove me nuts during his low T years, a close second was his lack of energy. The guy *shuffled* when he walked. He was tired all the time, and he did this thing where he *sighed* a lot. You know ... that thing that old folks do where they heave a great big sigh when they get up off the sofa?

This is an area where most men benefit once they start testosterone treatment. They rediscover energy, joy and a zest for life. It is always miraculous to me when I see it happen. Most of the time, they don't even realize how subdued they had become until they leave the low T fog behind. This was certainly the case with my husband. He went from couch potato to working out multiple times a week and starting a new martial art. It's like he's a different man!

## Improved Mood/Beating Depression

As I mentioned earlier, men with low testosterone are four times more likely to suffer from depression.

For many men with depression, starting on T treatment can improve mood, anxiety and ability to sleep. A review of 16 different studies involving a total of 944 men reported in the *Annals of Clinical Psychiatry* reached this conclusion:

> *"Testosterone may be used as a monotherapy in dysthymia (persistent mild depression) and minor depression or as an augmentation therapy in major depression in middle-aged hypogonadal men."*

The possibility that men can beat depression without resorting to anti-depressants with all their unpleasant side effects, including loss of libido, is very good news!

## Cognition and Memory

Your husband will most likely see an improvement in his ability to think and remember as the low T fog clears away. Healthy testosterone levels allow men to think and reason better, and are also associated with having better memory. Risk of Alzheimer's also goes down with higher testosterone levels.

For my husband, starting testosterone therapy meant that he stopped leaning on me to remember everyday things like how to get places and what the kids' schedules were. It was wonderful to have my sharp-witted guy back; I had missed him!

# Lean, Mean Fighting Machine

Okay, let's all just admit it. We *like* our guy to have muscles! Although we don't want him to turn into *The Hulk*, we also don't want him to be the Stay-Puft Marshmallow Man.

While he needs to work out and eat healthy, your husband can expect to see an improvement in his body composition once he starts T therapy. Higher levels of testosterone mean less fat and more muscle, a result consistently reported in multiple studies.

In one such study, men gained an average of more than six pounds of muscle after a year and a half of using testosterone gel. That's an amazing amount of muscle to add, especially since the men also lost about three pounds of fat during the same time period! That's where getting his testosterone back up to healthy levels is going to help.

# Improved Bone Density

Okay, bone density is not nearly as sexy as bigger muscles, but it's important. As I mentioned earlier, men with low testosterone levels have double the risk of getting osteoporosis. The good news is that testosterone therapy can actually increase bone density. While it doesn't happen overnight -- it can take upwards of a year to see improvement in spine and hipbone density -- multiple studies consistently show that continuous, long term testosterone therapy will eventually normalize bone density.

# General Health and Longevity

Too good to be true? Look at the conclusion that researchers reached after following a group of 3,690 men aged 70 to 89 in Australia from 2001 to 2004.

> *"Optimal circulating total testosterone is a robust biomarker for survival in aging men."*

While testosterone therapy is not the Fountain of Youth and it's not a substitute for living a healthy lifestyle, for a man with low T, testosterone treatment can provide the foundation for him to get his life and his health back on track.

## Benefits of Healthy T Levels

| |
|---|
| Increased Libido |
| Better Erections |
| Increased Energy and a Zest for Life |
| Improved Mood/Beating Depression |
| Improved Focus and Ability to Think Clearly |
| Improved Bone Density |
| Increased Muscle Mass & Decrease in Fat |
| Improved health |

Table 11

# What to Expect at this Point

- *You'll probably see at least a slight uptick in sexual frequency. He'll still be unsure of himself and hesitant to initiate.*

- *Morning erections may return. That provides a tremendous boon to his confidence.*

- *His energy and moods will improve. It's as if that layer of doom and gloom gets cleared away.*

- *If he's working out, he'll most likely see some muscle gains.*

- *It may become easier for him to lose fat, particularly in his abs.*

# Action Steps

- *Have realistic expectations. He's not going to become a wild caveman overnight.*
- *Encourage his first sexual attempts.*
- *Provide positive affirmation on his new changes.*

*I moaned and pushed upward, wanting more intensity. I was getting close, but he seemed to be holding back. He thrust a few more times, but it was a half-hearted effort.*

*"What's the matter?" I asked.*

*"Nothing. I … just … nothing," he said, and I realized that he had lost his erection.*

*Again.*

*I lay there, wanting to scream with frustration, but not wanting to make him feel bad. I knew he couldn't help it, but it was so tough to get so close … once again … only to have it all fizzle out.*

*I also worried about whether this was normal for a guy his age. I had heard that ED could indicate cardiovascular problems; I wondered whether something was really wrong with him.*

# Chapter 14
# If the Penis ain't Happy, ain't *Nobody* Happy
## *Dealing with Sexual Dysfunction*

I mentioned in the last chapter that testosterone therapy improves erectile dysfunction for roughly 60 percent of the men with low testosterone who are struggling with this problem.  Unfortunately, that still leaves 40 percent who can't get or maintain the erections they need for good sex. If you and your husband are in that remaining 40 percent, you know what a problem that is!

Often, ED goes beyond simply being a physical problem. The years of ED have affected both his confidence ... *and yours*. To treat ED effectively, you have to look at the psychological components as well as the physiological. Luckily, there are things you can do to address both issues.

In this chapter, we'll cover the mechanics of erections, how likely it is that T therapy will fix his ED, alternative therapies for those cases where testosterone treatment isn't enough, and how to address the confidence issues that are making the problem worse.

## Erections and Arousal are *Not* the Same

Erectile dysfunction is devastating to most men. As I stated earlier in the book, he feels that if his penis is broke, *he's* broke. An often-overlooked part of the equation, though, is that if his penis is broke, you may feel like *you're* broke. Most women in a low T marriage already struggle with feelings of self-doubt and rejection. When his penis doesn't get hard when he touches you, it just reinforces all those doubts in your mind. We women tend to equate erections with desire; however, while the two are related, they're not the same thing.

While you may understand this intellectually, knowing it is different than feeling it. You may understand logically that he can desire you and still not get hard, but if you're like many women, you haven't internalized that fact.

From the time a woman becomes sexually active, she learns to associate a guy's erection with his desire. When you first got married, the rules were simple. Touch his penis and he gets hard. Kiss him and he gets hard, smile at him and he gets hard, walk in the room and he gets hard. Hardness abounds! All of this lovely hardness served to not only reassure you that he found you attractive, it also strengthened your sense that erections equal arousal.

But nowadays, erections are scarce on the ground. Smiles, touches and kisses don't do the trick anymore. In fact, you can jump on top of him stark naked and an erection is still somewhat iffy. Something you both always took for granted has become a very big deal and you've started doubting whether he is still attracted to you. If you're like many women, you're wondering, "What's wrong with me?"

You need to realize that there's nothing wrong with you. The fact of the matter is that a man can feel very attracted and even aroused and still not get an erection. To understand why, you have to understand the structure of the penis and the mechanics of erections.

## The Structure of the Penis

The penis consists of a narrow central tube called the **urethra** (the tube through which urine and semen flow) covered by three spongy cylinders. The cylinder that contains the urethra is known as the **corpus spongiosum** and lies on the bottom of the penis; the other two cylinders lie on the top and sides and are filled with spongy tissue that engorges with blood during an erection.

The chambers that engorge with blood are called the **corpus cavernosum**, which always reminds me of a spell out of a *Harry Potter* book. I can just picture Hermione flicking her wand and commanding, "*Amplio corpus cavernosum!*" Too bad it's not that easy in real life.

163

A membrane called the **tunica albuginea** surrounds these three cylinders, and the whole package is covered by skin that moves freely over the structure.

While the penis is **flaccid** (soft or hanging loosely), the three cylinders contain only enough blood to keep the tissues supplied with nutrition; however, when the penis becomes erect, it contains eight times the amount of blood. Now, *that's* impressive! What miracle causes blood volume in the penis to increase by 800 percent?

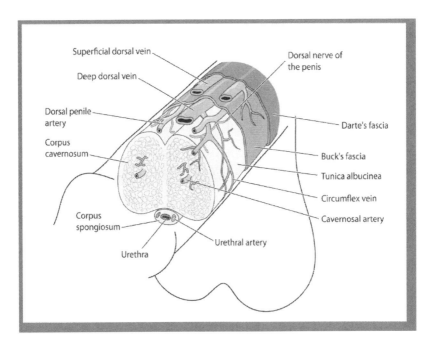

## The Mechanics of Erections

For couples who haven't experienced ED, erections seem as simple as breathing; however, they're actually incredibly complex with multiple moving parts and stages where things can go wrong.

It all starts in the brain where chemicals are released and travel down the spinal cord to special nerve cells in the penis. These nerves release nitric oxide which allows the smooth muscle tissue in the corpus cavernosum to relax and arteries to dilate, allowing more blood to flow in and become trapped in the spongy tissue of the corpus cavernosum.

This in turn constricts the veins against the surrounding tissue, preventing the blood from flowing back out, kind of like when you step on a garden hose to keep the water from flowing out. When certain nerves are stimulated, the muscles within the cavernosa contract, causing the erection to become full and hard. Of course, it's more complex than that, but that is enough detail for our general purposes.

In this chapter, we'll focus on three main factors involved in erectile problems:

- The effect low T has on physiological factors
- The effect low T has on psychological factors
- The effect factors *other* than testosterone are playing in the process

You can liken erections to a car engine. Hundreds of things can go wrong in between you turning the key and the engine actually starting, and it can be extremely difficult to isolate the problem. Or problems, for that matter, as it's quite possible to have multiple breakdowns in the process.

In the same way, hundreds of things can go wrong in the erection process, in between him having a sexual thought and his penis actually getting hard.

## How Low T Affects Physiological Factors

First of all, the genital region and sex organs are loaded with testosterone receptors, and testosterone works on all the sexual organs such as the penis, testicles, vas deferens, and even the prostate.

While there are multiple parts that have to work together to produce erections, you can group them into three main systems.

- *Nervous system* – Sends signals and activates nerve cells
- *Vascular system* – Supplies the blood necessary for erections
- *Muscular system* – Muscles in the pelvic region provide structural support necessary to maintain erections

As it turns out, testosterone plays a role in *all three of these systems*. For example, remember how it's chemical signals that control blood flow that cause erections? It's actually testosterone that directs those signals. In addition, testosterone affects the ability of veins to dilate enough to produce erections. Once you know all this, it becomes easier to understand why low testosterone has such a devastating effect on erections.

When a man is castrated, his body greatly reduces testosterone production; in addition, he almost completely loses his ability to have erections. At one time, it was thought by the medical community that this was because of a reduced sex drive. However, some interesting information came to light when scientists examined castrated rats.

A castrated rat produces fewer of the chemical signals necessary for erections and his body quickly loses the ability to produce them. In addition, the muscles that support the erection also weaken and atrophy. However, if you inject him with external testosterone, even months later, his body eventually restores the damaged nerves and muscle, and his ability to have erections is completely restored.

When another group of scientists studied castrated rabbits, they found that fat cells had replaced the smooth muscle cells in the corpus cavernosum, decreasing its ability to trap blood. This tells us that there are physiological factors at play when a man has deficient testosterone levels in addition to the psychological factors that prevent erections.

From studies like these and some human studies, we know that the systems most closely involved with the production of erections- the nervous system, the vascular system, and the muscular system - are all testosterone-dependent and are weakened by its absence. However, the good news is that we also know that testosterone can restore function fairly efficiently, not all of the time, but a great deal of the time.

## How Low T Affects Psychological Factors

What all of this information means is that there's a double whammy at play with low testosterone because in addition to affecting the actual physical mechanics of erections, low T also lowers the libido necessary to get the process started in the first place. Remember I told you that it all starts in the brain. Well, when libido disappears because T levels are low, there's nothing to trigger that initial surge in the brain causing it to release the neurotransmitters necessary for erections.

## Take Heart and Be Patient

If your husband has suffered from low testosterone for any length of time, it's very possible that it's affected the systems in his body that produce erections *in addition to* affecting his libido. It's also very possible that starting T therapy will help restore both the missing libido *plus* repair the mechanics. However, as Eugene Shippen, MD, points out in his book, *The Testosterone Syndrome*, testosterone replacement is not an immediate fix; it can't produce immediate erections like Viagra. Rather, it's a hormone that makes it possible for the body to rebuild its own process, but this takes time.

## Factors Other than Testosterone that Affect Erections

In addition to low testosterone, there are other factors that can cause ED, some of them controllable and some of them not.

- *Vascular conditions including high blood pressure* are the most common causes of ED. Conversely, ED can also be an indicator of vascular problems, and tends to precede coronary artery disease by three to five years.

Ironically enough, while high blood pressure itself can cause ED, so can some of the high blood pressure meds. There are some blood pressure meds, though, that not only don't hurt erections, they actually help. If your husband starts on a blood pressure med, he needs to be sure to ask his doctor which ones are 'erection-friendly'.

- ***Diabetes*** and ED are closely linked. 35-50% of men with diabetes have ED, and roughly half of them will be impotent by the time they hit 50.

In addition, ED can be an early indicator of having diabetes. Diabetes causes not only nerve damage, but also damages blood vessels. Now that you understand the role that nerves and blood vessels have in erectile function, you can see how this has a significant impact on ED.

- ***Hormonal Issues*** including low testosterone, high or low estrogen, thyroid problems, elevated prolactin, pituitary dysfunction, etc.

It's worth noting here that just as testosterone does, estrogen also plays an important role in erections. Your husband's doctor needs to make sure that estrogen levels are optimal.

- ***Lifestyle Factors*** such as drugs, alcohol, smoking, prescription and over-the-counter meds, and sleep deprivation all take a toll on erections.

> *One common over-the-counter med is notorious for causing ED.*
>
> *Pseudoephedrine, an ingredient in some decongestants, is a vasoconstrictor sometimes used to treat priapism (erection that won't go away).*

Some prescription meds that commonly affect erections include anti-depressants, certain blood pressure meds, and cholesterol-lowering meds, to name a few.

- **Infections or pelvic trauma** from prostate, colon or bladder surgery can damage the nerves and blood vessels involved in erections.

- **Performance anxiety and other psychological issues** can be factors.

- **Neurological conditions** such as Multiple Sclerosis, Parkinson's disease and Alzheimer's disease normally cause ED problems.

As an aside, it's interesting to note that the first two factors, vascular conditions and diabetes, are responsible for the vast majority of erectile difficulties, and both are much more common when testosterone levels are inadequate. As I mentioned earlier, men with low T are twice as likely to have cardiovascular disease and four times as likely to have diabetes.

Thus, testosterone levels have a significant impact on erections, both directly and indirectly.

# Beyond T Therapy - Fixing the ED

Okay, we know that low T is not the only thing, or even the main thing, that causes ED. It's great when T therapy is enough to resolve a guy's ED, but what happens if your husband is in that group for whom T therapy *isn't* enough? Because let's be candid here ... while there are a lot of work-arounds you can do when his penis isn't working, honestly, sometimes you just need a good hard pounding! Are the two of you simply out of luck?

The bad news about ED is that between 15 and 30 million men in the US struggle with it, with almost half of all men between ages 40 to 70 experiencing at least occasional ED. The good news is that having such a large group of potential customers means that the drug companies have been very busy coming up with ED treatments that are quite effective.

There are actually a lot of fixes for ED, and they go beyond simply Viagra, Cialis and Levitra, but let's start there as the first-line option.

## *The Triumphant Triumvirate*

Cialis, Viagra and Levitra all belong to a group of prescription meds called PDE-5 inhibitors. The PDE-5 inhibitors enhance the effects of nitric oxide in dilating the blood vessels, which relaxes the smooth muscle tissue in the corpus cavernosum, allowing the penis to fill with blood.

While Cialis, Viagra and Levitra all do basically the same thing, there are some key differences that may determine which one is best for you and your husband.

Cialis is a favorite for a lot of guys because it lasts so much longer than either Viagra or Levitra. Whereas Viagra and Levitra both last for about four hours, Cialis lasts for roughly 36. This allows for a lot more spontaneity, which means that if sex doesn't work out during a particular time period, there's not that sinking feeling of "Oh, I just wasted a lot of money on a pill I didn't even use." Taking Viagra or Levitra with food can decrease absorption and make them less effective, whereas food consumption doesn't seem to affect Cialis, again allowing for more spontaneity.

All three are available in different strengths, and it usually takes a bit of tweaking to get the dosage right. There are also daily dose versions of Cialis available that are good options for some men.

Being able to get good erections again has a tremendous impact on a man's confidence.

*"I had forgotten what it's like to have a real erection. I had gotten so used to my penis only going to a 90 degree angle that I forgot it used to go all the way up to 45 degrees!"*

*--Michael, 42, IT Specialist*

## Side Effects and Drug Interactions

Cialis, Viagra and Levitra all have common side effects including congestion, flushing, and sometimes headaches and heartburn. With Cialis, he can also have some aches and pains in his back. In addition, less commonly, a guy can experience vision problems that generally go away when he stops use. Most of the guys I've worked with have tolerated the side effects fairly well.

As with any medicine, there are certain people who need to be cautious about using ED drugs. Because they can slightly lower blood pressure, they might be a problem for guys who already have low blood pressure. While men who are taking meds for high blood pressure are generally okay to use ED meds, guys who have uncontrolled hypertension (high blood pressure), or who have had a recent heart attack or stroke may not be good candidates.

In addition, ED meds can interact with other meds, including the ones listed below, with serious results. Obviously, your husband needs to talk to his doctor about any meds he's taking prior to getting a prescription.

- *Nitrates*
- *HIV protease inhibitors*
- *Some antibiotics*
- *Other ED meds*
- *Alpha-blockers and some other blood pressure meds*

## New Kids on the Block

There are two fairly new PDE-5 inhibitors now available in addition to the big three; Stendra and Staxyn. They are similar to the other three, but Stendra starts working quicker, within about 15 minutes, and can last up to five hours. Staxyn has the same active ingredient as Levitra but dissolves on the tongue; since it bypasses the digestive system, it has the potential to take effect more quickly than Levitra tablets.

## The Low T – ED Loop

While it's obvious how the ED meds improve the physiological component of ED, it's not as immediately apparent how they can also work on the psychological component.

As I mentioned earlier in the chapter, when a man struggles with erectile problems for any length of time, it has a huge impact on his confidence levels. Because sex has turned into such an anxious and embarrassing experience, his libido decreases. This creates a negative loop that looks like the one below:

| Low T - ED Loop |
| --- |
| Low T → Loss of erections<br><br>Loss of erections → Performance Anxiety → Loss of libido |

One thing that can help break this cycle is for a guy to use one of the ED drugs long enough to alleviate his performance anxiety. I've worked with couples where the husband's libido increased before he ever took the first dose of testosterone simply because he started using Cialis, et al. Losing the performance anxiety was enough to break the negative loop and help him feel confident enough to want sex again. Talk about instant results!

## The Spirit is Willing

A wife's attitude about her husband using an ED med has a major impact on whether he feels comfortable with it. Many women struggle with the idea that he 'needs a drug' in order to get 'turned on' for sex. It's important to understand that it doesn't work like that. Cialis and Viagra don't *create* desire. A man still has to have the sexual impulse that prompts the chemical messengers to travel down the spine and start the whole erection process. The PDE-5 inhibitors simply keep the process from derailing at the point where nitric oxide is released.

You need to remember that his lack of erections doesn't mean a lack of desire. It's important to internalize this because the more comfortable you are with the idea of him taking Cialis, et al., the more comfortable he'll be taking it. Most guys are already embarrassed by needing an ED med; if there's tension between the two of you over it, he's never going to use it ... and you're never going to get the sex you want!

It's also important to realize that him using an ED med isn't necessarily a forever thing. What I've seen happen fairly often is that a guy will start using an ED med around the same time he starts T therapy. His erections start coming back and he gains confidence. Over time, as he starts working out and gets more fit, he can often actually cut back on the ED drug and still have great erections. Once he breaks that *Low T - ED loop* I mentioned earlier, *and* gets a good level of testosterone in his system, he can sometimes eliminate the need for the ED med altogether. But he's going to need your encouragement and support to get there.

## Radioactive Poison?

If you're like many women, in addition to the concern that he needs a drug to turn him on, one of the things that makes you uncomfortable about ED drugs is that you have no idea what's actually in them.

I was initially freaked out about the idea of my husband taking a pill that would give him an erection. I think I had some kind of idea that he was ingesting radioactive poison that would change him from Bruce Banner to *The Hulk*. It was immensely reassuring to me when I did the research into the ED meds and actually learned how they work in the body.

Viagra was the first PDE-5 inhibitor to be developed. A team of researchers at Pfizer's Labs in Sandwich, England, was working on a drug - then known as UK-92480 - that selectively blocked an enzyme called PDE-5 (phosphodiesterase type 5). They hoped that blocking this enzyme would allow blood vessels to expand and have a positive effect on angina. While it only had a moderate effect on angina, volunteers were reporting an interesting side effect – increased erections. The rest, of course, is history.

Since then, the active ingredient in Viagra, sildenafil, has been tested and used for multiple conditions other than ED, including heart failure in adults, pulmonary hypertension in children, underdeveloped hearts in kids and young adults, and chronic lung disease in premature babies, amongst others.

In fact, recent research has led some doctors to recommend that Viagra be used by some at-risk patients to prevent heart attacks and strokes. These researchers have found that Viagra can substantially improve men's cardiac function and that men with heart failure who also used Viagra had hearts that worked more efficiently.

Daily use Cialis has been shown to help symptoms of benign prostatic hyperplasia (BPH) and is also approved for the treatment of pulmonary hypertension.

While ED drugs *can* be a problem for men with certain health issues, and they *can* interact with certain medications, for the vast majority of men who use them they are safe. In fact, for certain men, they may actually enhance health.

---

## Buying Cialis without Breaking the Bank

One of the problems with Cialis, et al., is that they are so expensive.

Because of this, your husband may want to try ordering a generic version from an on-line pharmacy; many men find this to be much more affordable. He just needs to make sure it is legal to do so in his region and that the pharmacy is reputable and requires a prescription.

His doctor may have free samples your husband can try, and the makers of Cialis also offer a coupon on their website for a free month's supply. He simply prints it off and presents it to his local pharmacy along with his prescription.

---

## When Viagra Doesn't Work

PDE-5 inhibitors are effective for up to 85% of the men who use them, depending on the dosage used. For the guy in that remaining 15%, however, having Viagra fail is often a devastating experience. He's pinned all his hopes of reclaiming his sex life on Viagra, only to have them dashed. He often feels that Viagra was his last resort and that he's out of options

This isn't the case, however. While Cialis, et al., are the first-line options for ED, if they're not effective, there are second-line options he can try that are quite effective for most men.

Most of the second-line ED treatments involve injectable meds, although there is also a topical gel available in some areas.

## Injectable Meds

Quite a few prescription meds achieve very good results when injected directly into the penis. Like the PDE-5 inhibitors, they work by relaxing the smooth muscles and widening the blood vessels in the penis. Unlike the PDE-5 inhibitors, however, they are not dependent on nerve stimulation, so they produce an erection even with minimal sexual stimulation.

It's a shame that the injectable meds are not as well known or advertised as Cialis, et al. because once you get past the initial *ouch* factor, the injectables have a lot to recommend them, especially for men who don't respond to the PDE-5 inhibitors.

The biggest disadvantage, of course, is that they must be injected directly into the penis; however, the needle used is quite small and fine-gauged, and the amount of medicine injected is minimal. The injections *can* cause pain, bruising and -- if injected too frequently or in the same spot -- scarring, but for the most part, are well tolerated by many men.

### Advantages of Injectables
- *They produce very strong erections.*
- *They require only minimal stimulation to be effective.*
- *Men whose medical conditions or medications prevent them from using a PDE-5 inhibitor can sometimes use them.*

### Disadvantages of Injectables
- *Must be injected*
- *Can cause pain, bruising or scarring if injected too frequently or in the same spot*

Injectables can be a single med or a combination of meds put together by a compounding pharmacy. The compounds tend to work together to be more effective than a single med, and are effective at smaller doses, thus decreasing side effects. Some common injectables and combinations include:

- *Phentolamine – called* Regitine
- *Alprostadil – called* Caverject
- *Papaverine + phentolamine – called* Bi-Mix
- *Papaverine + phentolamine + Alprostadil – called* Trimix *(a very effective combination for most men)*
- *Papaverine + phentolamine + Alprostadil + Atropine – called* Quad-Mix *(a good option for men in whom* Trimix *wasn't effective)*

## Important Warning: Priapism

One of the most dangerous side effects of most of the injectables is the potential for priapism, an erection that won't subside. While this may sound like a good thing to you at the moment, priapism can actually permanently damage a man's penis because the blood is trapped inside the corpus cavernosum and loses oxygen, destroying the tissue in the penis. An erection that lasts for more than four hours is dangerous and is an emergency that requires medical treatment.

To decrease the possibility of priapism, the injectable meds should never be used with the PDE-5 inhibitors without a doctor's okay. The combination of the two makes priapism more likely.

## Alprostadil

One of the injectables, Alprostadil, is also available as a pellet called Muse that's inserted into the urethra. In addition, it's recently become available in Canada as a topical gel called Vitaros that's applied to the penis. At the time of writing, Alprostadil gel was pending approval in the US.

The injectable form is the most effective with a higher than 80% success rate. The topical gel is next at 60-70%, and the pellet form comes in last with a success rate of 30-40%.

Even though the topical gel is somewhat less effective than the injectable form of Alprostadil, it may still be a good option for those men who need more than Viagra but aren't crazy about the idea of injecting into their penis or inserting into their urethra.

The topical gel doesn't seem to have any serious side effects, but most men get a warming sensation for five to twenty minutes after applying it, with roughly 20% saying that they actually experienced some discomfort.

One concern many men have about Alprostadil topical gel is whether it's safe to have intercourse with their wife after they've applied the gel. Studies haven't shown any problematic side effects for the woman; in fact, in one study, researchers tested Alprostadil gel on women to see how it affected blood flow in the genital region. All the women in the study had labial and clitoral engorgement, and 72% reported a 'pleasant sensation of warmth', with no systemic side effects.

## Strengthening the Muscles

An often-overlooked method of improving ED is simply strengthening the pelvic floor muscles that support erections. While this obviously doesn't have the immediate impact that ED meds do, it can be surprisingly effective.

Some studies have shown that strengthening the pelvic floor muscles through exercise is almost as effective as using some of the ED meds, with 40% of the men regaining full function, and an additional 30-35% of the men showing at least some improvement.

The muscles in the pelvic region are packed with testosterone receptors and are extremely dependent on adequate testosterone levels to function properly. As your husband's T levels went down, these muscles declined and atrophied, with the muscle fibers actually thinning. Now that his T levels are optimal again, he needs to rebuild those muscles by doing exercises called Kegels to strengthen them. Yup, these are basically the same Kegels you do to strengthen your own pelvic floor muscles.

It's important that he do kegels effectively in order to get results. The Internet is loaded with sites that explain how to do them and YouTube has some great videos on the topic if you search 'man kegels'.

While your guy may not be particularly thrilled to do Kegels, I suspect you'll get his attention after you explain the key benefits:

- *Stronger erections*
- *More-powerful orgasms*
- *More-powerful ejaculations*
- *Ability to last longer*
- *Improvement of incontinence issues like dribbling and leaks*

If that's not enough to get him squeezing, I don't know what will!

## *Other Options*

For those guys for whom none of the above works, the next step is a visit to a urologist who specializes in erectile dysfunction. There are a number of different tests that can evaluate where the problem or problems lie, including ultrasounds that check the condition of penile arteries, blood flows and leaks, any scarring of the tissue that might be causing problems, etc.

There's also a test called an NPT (nocturnal penile tumescence) test that uses special gauges to see whether erections are happening during sleep; this helps separate physiological from psychological causes.

| Drugs that Help ED |
|---|
| **PDE-5 Inhibitors**<br>• *Viagra*<br>• *Cialis*<br>• *Levitra*<br>• *Stendra*<br>• *Staxyn* |
| **Injectables**<br>• *Phentolamine (*Regitine*)*<br>• *Alprostadil (*Caverject*)*<br>• *Papaverine + phentolamine* (Bi-Mix*)*<br>• *Papaverine + phentolamine + Alprostadil (*Trimix*)*<br>• *Papaverine, Phentolamine, Alprostadil, Atropine (*Quad-Mix*)* |
| **Alprostadil**<br><br>• *Pellet (Muse)*<br>• *Topical gel (available as* Vitaros *in Canada; pending approval in the US)* |

Table 12

There are also treatments like vacuum pump devices and surgical options for when nothing else works, so if your husband is not responding to first or second-line options, don't give up hope. Set up an appointment with a good urologist and keep working to find your answers.

## Canary in the Coal Mine

The last thing I'll discuss in this chapter is possibly the most important. While ED has a significant impact on your sex life, there are far deeper implications than simply sex. As I mentioned earlier, ED can be one of the first warning signs of cardiovascular problems. I don't mean to scare you, but men who have ED - even when they initially show no signs of heart problems - are much more likely to eventually experience significant cardiovascular events, usually within the next three to five years.

The human heart has more testosterone receptors than any other muscle in the body and low testosterone levels are strongly associated with cardiovascular health. Testosterone stimulates nitric oxide which acts as a vasodilator and is essential not only for strong erections, but also for a healthy heart and healthy blood vessels.

If your husband's ED doesn't resolve after his T levels get stable and after working on his pelvic floor muscles, it's time to get into a cardiologist. It could literally save his life!

## The Foundation

The main take-away I hope you get from this chapter is that just like low testosterone, ED is a medical issue and there are solutions available. While his lack of erections feels personal to you, it's not. You simply have to fix the medical in order to move forward.

Getting his penis working again provides a foundation for moving on to *Stage Four – Restoring the Marriage*. It's vital to address his ED issues in order to restore your husband's confidence … and yours.

# What to Expect at this Point

- *If your husband has experienced ED during the low T years, it's affected both of your confidence levels. You are probably wondering whether he still finds you attractive; he probably feels like less than a man.*
- *His performance anxiety has probably decreased his libido.*
- *T therapy may gradually improve his ED, but it won't be immediate.*

- *He may be resistant to the idea of using Cialis, et al., because it feels emasculating.*
- *The idea of him using ED meds may seem scary.*
- *You worry that his ED indicates a larger health issue.*

# Action Steps

- *Understand that he can be aroused by you and still not get hard.*
- *Recognize that ED is frustrating and humiliating to him.*
- *You may feel frustrated when his penis doesn't work; try to be matter-of-fact about it. Stay as positive and encouraging as possible.*
- *Talk to him about the pros and cons of Cialis, et al.*
- *Encourage him to ask his doctor about trying an ED med, and to ask the doctor for samples.*
- *Check to see if your insurance covers any of the meds.*
- *Stay away from websites where they will sell you 'Viagra' without a prescription. There's simply no way to know what you're getting.*
- *If first-line ED meds aren't working, don't lose hope. There are second-line meds that will most likely do the trick.*
- *If the ED doesn't eventually resolve, encourage your husband to see a cardiologist and/or urologist to look for underlying health issues.*

# Stage Four

# Restoring Your Low T Marriage

*"If you've changed your mind about wanting sex, will you just go ahead and tell me so I can get on with my evening?" I asked, cutting my husband off in mid-sentence.*

*His voice had been droning on in my ears, talking about how we were going to get our relationship back on track, how much he loved me, how attractive I was, and on and on.*

*"What?" he asked, surprised by my interruption.*

*He did this a lot ... talked about how attractive I was ... how sexy I was ... how much he wanted to make love to me ... but that's all it was ...* **talk**.

*There was always a reason he didn't initiate. He was too tired from work, he wasn't sure if I was interested, he was sore from working out, he was waiting for the kids to go to bed, blah blah blah. Same story, different day.*

*He had been talking about sex all day long, telling me how much he wanted me and how he couldn't wait to take me to bed. When he left for his martial arts class, he told me to get ready to be ravished when he got home.*

*However, by the time he got home, wet with sweat, he was exhausted. He showered and ate and by 9:30, he was ready for bed. It was obvious that sex was the furthest thing from his mind.*

*"You said earlier that you wanted sex, so if you've changed your mind, just come out and tell me," I replied.*

*"Oh ..... no, I wasn't planning on sex," he said. "I thought we would just snuggle for a little bit and then have an early night."*

*"Okay, thanks for letting me know," I said, my heart heavy as I left the room.*

# Chapter 15
# Happily Ever After?
## *Rewiring the Circuits*

When my husband first started testosterone treatment, we assumed that once he fixed his hormones, our problems were solved and we were done; however, it didn't happen quite like that. Our sex life simply wasn't bouncing back the way we had expected it to. Instead, we started on a nearly two-year journey of relearning to be a couple again. It was at times more frustrating *after* he started T therapy than before it. We didn't know what to 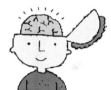 expect and there were no resources out there to help us. Trust me; I looked for them.

This is the point where we almost lost hope. After all, if we had done all this work to figure out a solution to the original mystery of his missing libido only to find that his libido was still missing, then what was there left to try? We were both confused and frustrated.

In working with low T couples, I've learned that this stage is also simply part of the process. It's predictable and solvable. You just have to understand what's going on.

There are three main reasons why a couple's sex life doesn't immediately bounce back after T therapy:

- *Low T changes a man's neural pathways.*
- *Low T affects more than just the general hormone system.*
- *Low T changes the dynamics in the marriage.*

## Why Testosterone Isn't a Magic Bullet

So if the problem was low T, and now he's getting testosterone treatment and the labs say his numbers are right ... why isn't everything better?

Well, let's clarify that. Testosterone treatment has fixed some things, but while his energy and mood have improved, the sex really ... *hasn't*. Maybe he's showing a bit more interest and you occasionally see that certain glint in his eye, but he still doesn't really initiate all that often and it seems like he can take it or leave it. Even though your husband's hormone levels are finally stable, he still doesn't seem to have that high desire he used to have. What's up with that?

Maybe he's just not a sexual person anymore. Or is he? Well ... it's complicated.

## Low T Affects Neural Pathways

For those men who have had low testosterone levels for a long time, their brain patterns have actually changed. Brain development depends on the experiences you have. Electrical activity in different areas of the brain shapes the way the brain circuits develop. The circuits that get used the most often are the ones that grow more developed, the ones that are rarely used become weaker, and are eventually pruned away. Scientists have a term for this, "Cells that fire together, wire together."

> *Sex drive is a function of hormones + brain circuitry. Your guy has some catching up to do.*

Do you see where I'm going with this? Even though his hormone levels are now fixed, the brain circuitry that would support a healthy libido has atrophied. Now does his behavior make more sense to you?

The bad news is that fixing the hormones is not necessarily an immediate fix for your sex life. The good news is that there are specific things you can both do that will help his brain develop the neural pathways that support a healthy libido. While in the past you may have felt powerless to do anything about your husband's lack of sexual desire, now that his hormones are fixed, it's a whole new ball game.

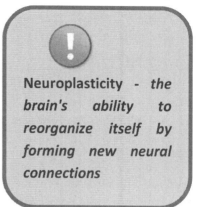

**Neuroplasticity - *the brain's ability to reorganize itself by forming new neural connections***

Even though you can't instantly repair the neural pathways, there are things you *can* do that will create an environment conducive to healing.

## Neuroplasticity – or How Do You Change Your Brain?

*Neuroplasticity* is a term that refers to the fact that changes in the neural pathways in the brain are possible due to changes in behavior, environment, thinking, emotions, hormones, and nutrition. This is a rapidly growing field and more and more studies are starting to expand our knowledge of what is possible. What we currently know is based on both animal and human studies. While the information is still coming in and the body of knowledge is incomplete, there are some key factors that have been shown to increase the rate at which you can change your brain patterns. The best part is that these factors aren't really all that complicated, they simply take a bit of effort.

*Intense Exercise* seems to be the single-most effective way to encourage neuroplasticity, and it doesn't much matter what type. Running, interval training, yoga, or Cross Fit will all do the trick. You just need to move enough to release the endorphins that support brain development.

***Reduced Stress*** is critical. Quite simply, stress reduces your brain's ability to change, and it seems that the more severe and prolonged the stress is, the more difficult it is to develop new neural pathways.

***Sufficient sleep*** increases your brain's ability to repair itself. As close to eight hours of sleep as possible is optimal.

***An enriched environment*** seems to spur neuroplasticity as well. What does that mean, exactly? Well, for rats, it means more tunnels, mazes and exercise wheels in their cages. For children, it means a plethora of objects that stimulate curiosity and learning and give tactile and olfactory stimulus. In other words, our world needs to be full of things that are interesting, and look, feel and smell good.

***Limited calorie restriction*** also seems to play a role. At first glance, this seems counter-intuitive. It would seem to make more sense that people who are well-fed are better able to reorganize their neural pathways; however, short-term calorie restriction provides just enough stress in the body to spur brain development.

In addition to short-term calorie restriction, there are certain things you can include in your diet that will improve your brain's ability to change. These include:

- ***Omega-3 fatty acids***, available in supplement form or through food sources including fish and some nuts and seeds
- ***Flavonoids*** found in blueberries, raspberries, green tea, and dark chocolate, amongst others

***Sunlight***, in addition to providing necessary Vitamin D, also increases neuroplasticity. It doesn't take much, a short exposure of about ten minutes to the face has a positive effect.

***Rewarding experiences*** are also thought to help.

***Optimal levels of testosterone and estrogen*** increase the brain's ability to develop new neurons.

***Engaging in sexual thoughts and behaviors*** increases the sexual pathways in the brain. Hence, sex begets more sex.

Engaging in these activities will help the two of you develop the foundations that support sexuality. Changing neural pathways is only one part of the solution, however. In order to understand what you need to do to get your marriage back on track, you also need to understand exactly how the brain is wired for love, attraction and sex.

# Low T Affects More Than Just the General Hormone System

Low testosterone is a unique medical issue in that it not only affects a man's health; it also affects his sex drive. And sex is an extremely personal issue. With other medical issues ... say, an injured leg ... it is clear that the medical problem has nothing to do with you as a woman. However, as a woman and a wife, it is tough to separate out your husband's libido ... or lack of it ... from his feelings of attraction for you. These are two closely related issues, and they tend to blur together in your mind. But libido and attraction are two separate things and are influenced by different hormones and neurotransmitters.

## *The Three Love Systems*

Helen Fisher, PhD, a renowned biological anthropologist and Senior Research Fellow for The Kinsey Institute, has laid out three separate, but interrelated love systems that affect romantic love. These systems, influenced by different hormones and neurotransmitters in the body, are responsible for different feelings.

- **The Dopamine system** creates feelings of attraction and excitement.
- **The Oxytocin system** causes feelings of being attached and bonded.
- **The General Hormone system** is fueled primarily by testosterone and estrogen, and impacts libido.

**Attraction** occurs when a couple first meet and fall in love, and powerful changes occur in the brain. These changes involve dopamine 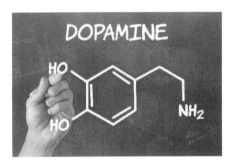 centers in the brain and can actually be seen on an MRI. Dopamine is a neurotransmitter that creates feelings of bliss, pleasure, and euphoria. When they 'fall in love', people experience feelings of exhilaration, excitement, focused attention on the romantic partner, and a craving to be with each other.

**Attachment** develops as the relationship deepens, and couples start having feelings of being bonded or attached to each other. They have feelings of calm, peace, and security when they're with each other. These feelings are caused by oxytocin in women, and oxytocin/vasopressin in men.

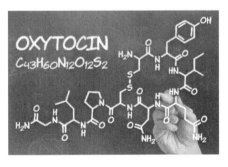

Oxytocin has been called the bonding hormone. We produce this hormone when we engage in activities that make us feel closer to someone. It causes feelings of trust and comfort. Women produce copious amounts of oxytocin when they breastfeed a baby; people produce oxytocin when they touch each other.

*General Hormones* comprise the third love system, which is the general drive to have sex, either alone or with a partner, powered primarily by testosterone and estrogen.

The three love systems operate together to create intense feelings of love and attraction between a man and woman. Here's the important thing to remember; when one of the systems is affected, it disrupts a

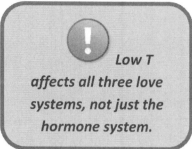

***Low T affects all three love systems, not just the hormone system.***

couple's relationship in real and lasting ways because it also puts stress on the other two love systems. Understanding this is key to repairing a low T marriage.

It's somewhat intuitive that low testosterone impacts general sex drive, but it's not as immediately clear how it also affects attraction and attachment. Let's take a look at that.

## Attraction, but Not Desire

Up until now, you've assumed that because your husband hasn't had sexual desire for you, it meant that he wasn't attracted to you. This is not necessarily the case and it's one of the most confusing parts of the process to understand.

During his low T years, my husband would frequently compliment my appearance and tell me how pretty I was. He acted as if he were attracted to me, but then bedtime would come without him initiating sex. I couldn't understand it. I wondered why, if he was attracted to me, he didn't follow up on that attraction.

What I didn't know then is that desire and attraction are not the same thing. They're related to each other and they influence each other, but they're two separate things. Sexual desire, or libido, is fueled by the general hormone system, while attraction is fueled by the dopamine system.

My husband wasn't being a hypocrite as I thought at the time; he actually was genuinely attracted to me. He simply didn't have the hormones to turn his attraction into sexual desire. He had attraction without desire.

## Desire, but Not Attraction

Now here's where it gets a bit tricky. You can also have desire, but not attraction. This is something that frequently confuses and creates

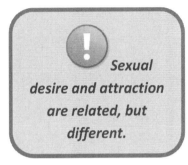

**Sexual desire and attraction are related, but different.**

guilt in women in a low T marriage. While they may feel sexual desire, they're very bothered by the fact that they aren't necessarily attracted to their low T husband.

At first glance, this doesn't seem to make sense. If she has a libido, why doesn't she want sex with her husband? Once you recognize that attraction and desire are fueled by two separate love systems, it becomes much more understandable. Her general hormone system is just fine and so she feels sexual desire, but the low T is taking a toll on the dopamine love system that fuels attraction.

## Low T Affects Attraction

Low testosterone can take a huge hit on a woman's attraction for her husband. The reasons for this become clear when you look at what masculine traits attract women. Women are attracted to men who are energetic, bold, and confident. We are also attracted to men who are physically fit and well-muscled. Remember I'm not talking about what makes you love a man, but what makes you actually sexually attracted to him. Other traits we find attractive are intelligence and the ability to be decisive. We are attracted to men who are leaders in their social group. Most importantly, we're attracted to men who not only have a strong desire for sex, but who are also able to physically carry through on that desire.

Now let's pull up that list of low T symptoms from Chapter One.

- *Low sex drive*
- *Low energy, easily fatigued*
- *Less fun, less social*
- *Difficulty in concentrating, forgetful*
- *Problems getting a strong erection that lasts*
- *Grumpy, stressed and moody*
- *Weight gain, particularly in his abdomen*
- *Muscle loss*

Do you begin to see the problem? Low T impacts the masculine traits that attract us. Through no fault of his own, while his testosterone was low, your husband acted in ways that were less attractive to you. As his behavior changed and your attraction for him diminished, it substantially changed your relationship dynamics.

## Low T Affects Attachment

Attachment is created by the oxytocin hormone, and refers to the feeling of being bonded or connected to your partner. Attachment comes about through having multiple interactions together; creating a home and family, spending time together, being in close proximity to each other, touching each other, 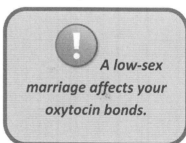 showing appreciation for each other, and in general, simply being warm and affectionate.

*A low-sex marriage affects your oxytocin bonds.*

What happens in a low T marriage, though, is that a couple gradually drifts apart. As the wife loses attraction for her husband, she starts treating him differently. She may become sharp and critical with him, or sometimes simply indifferent to him, which diminishes his feelings of comfort with her, and thus decreases attachment. As a result, he withdraws, further increasing the distance between the two of them. Throw in the fact that a guy with low T typically becomes less social in general, tending to isolate himself, and it becomes a fairly toxic mix.

The big kicker, though, in lowering attachment is the lack of sex. Wait, what does sex have to do with creating an oxytocin bond? It turns out that as two people touch and kiss each other, multiple mechanisms are triggered in the brain, releasing chemicals and neurotransmitters that lower stress and boost mood. Pleasure hormones also increase, leading to deep relaxation and a reduction in anxiety.

As we approach orgasm, neural circuits of pleasure, reward and emotion are activated. The hypothalamus releases the hormone oxytocin and it floods the brain and spinal cord, intensifying feelings of pleasure. Why is this important?

Oxytocin is one of the primary hormones responsible for bonding and trust in humans; it helps lower our defenses and allows us to trust people more, and it increases feelings of empathy and forgiveness. Oxytocin also increases our ability to remain positive during conflict and it decreases the stress hormone, cortisol, thus helping us handle conflict more easily. In a very real sense, oxytocin = love. As unromantic as it sounds, when you increase your oxytocin levels, you increase your feelings of love for your partner.

As Beth told me:

*"I don't really miss sex all that much but now that we've stopped having it, we seem to fight all the time. My husband is increasingly angry and resentful with me. I don't feel any sense of connection to him and it seems that the feeling is mutual. Every little decision has become this huge battle between the two of us."*

—Beth, 49, Hair Stylist

A sexless marriage is about a lot more than just orgasms. The act of having sex bonds and connects us in ways that last well beyond the encounter.

## *When One Love System Is Affected*

You're in a situation where the general hormone system has been damaged for a while and it's affected the other two love systems. It may seem overwhelming to both of you to regain your marriage. How do you fix it all? Where do you start?

The solution is to not only repair the general hormone system, but to also strengthen the other two systems that have been affected. This will be a substantial part of your recovery process.

# Low T Changes Your Marriage Dynamics

The last way in which low T changes your marriage is that the repeated sexual rejection over the years typically makes you hypersensitive to rejection. At the same time, the years of pressure to be more sexual than he's able to causes your husband to become highly reactive to sexual pressure. If you don't understand and repair this dynamic, it can create enormous problems in your recovery process.

## *You're Hypersensitive to Rejection*

Because men are typically the ones who pursue women, they tend to become accustomed to sexual rejection quite early in their lives, normally by their late teens. Women, on the other hand, are simply not used to sexual rejection. As a rule, while men control commitment, women control sex. A passably attractive woman usually has no dearth of potential sexual opportunities.

> *You're hypersensitive to rejection and he's highly reactive to sexual pressure.*

Chances are that you never experienced sexual rejection before your husband's sex drive went missing. You simply aren't equipped to deal with the level of rejection you've experienced during the low T years, and it's made you hypersensitive to rejection.

You interpret everything through this rejection lens. Rejection is a trigger for you, and over the years, your reactions have become more and more volatile. It may have gotten so bad by this point that the simplest thing can set you off. Maybe he faces his shoes east instead of west when he goes to bed, and everybody knows that this is the universal sign for not wanting sex. You go to bed seething, with him having no idea what's going on or what he's done wrong. You eventually explode and add yet more negative energy into an already difficult situation.

What you have to understand is that after a while, the pain of being rejected starts feeling *normal,* and it becomes your knee-jerk reaction even in situations where you're not actually being rejected. You end up with this repeating cycle of ever-increasing death spirals that create huge amounts of negative energy in your marriage and tank both attraction and attachment.

## He's Highly Reactive to Sexual Pressure

Here's the part you need to understand; the angrier you are, the less attractive he finds you and the more he withdraws. In the same way that you're reactive to rejection, your husband is reactive to the pressure to perform. Every time you push him for more sex, you make it more difficult for him to want sex. Your actions are putting you further and further from what you most want ... a satisfying sex life with your husband. The more pressure he feels that he *ought* to have sex, the less he's able to *want* to have sex. Sexual desire can't be forced. While having a temper tantrum may cause him to *have* sex with you, it will also keep him from *wanting* sex with you.

Overcoming both *your* hypersensitivity to rejection and *his* reactivity to sexual pressure is one of the more difficult challenges in the *Recovery Stage*, but once you understand what's going on, it becomes considerably easier.

# Marriage and Baseball

What in the world do they have in common? Well, I've found that when dealing with guys, it's helpful to use a sports metaphor to keep the process positive. So we're going to treat low T like it's an injury to a professional athlete.

If you think about it, low T and a sports injury can often look the same in terms of what guys *do*. Often an injured player denies that he's injured and just walks it off, hoping it gets better. But it's apparent to everyone around him that he needs help.

The doctor is called in against the player's protests and diagnoses a stress fracture. Everyone groans because they know it will be months before he's back in the game, but at least once he has a diagnosis, he knows what he's dealing with and what to do to heal. There's a predictable recovery process and this gives him hope. It's the same with a low T marriage. Knowing what to expect makes the whole process much easier.

Just like the baseball player who has been diagnosed and treated, you and your husband still have some rehab to do before you're back in the game. The *Recovery Stage* is when you'll do the repair work needed to heal your marriage.

# Three Step Recovery

In working with couples to help them recover their Low T marriage, I've found that it's helpful to break down the *Recovery Stage* into three separate steps:

- *Healing the Injury*
- *Cleared for Practice*
- *Getting Back in the Game*

These steps are fluid and there's some overlap, but each step is characterized by a different focus. Going through the recovery process systematically is how you will rebuild your marriage and find your way back to the sexual and emotional intimacy you crave. Mastering the challenges in one step helps prepare you to take on the challenges in the next. We'll talk about the different steps in detail in the next few chapters.

# What to Expect at This Point

- *Your sex life probably hasn't bounced back the way you thought it would now that his T levels are fixed.*
- *He 'talks' about sex more than he actually initiates, and it drives you nuts.*
- *He still seems sexually avoidant.*
- *You are increasingly volatile each time you feel sexually rejected.*
- *While you want sex, you may not be particularly attracted to him. While he seems attracted to you, he may not be particularly interested in sex.*
- *T levels are still stabilizing and you'll see some ups and downs for a while. This will eventually smooth out.*

# Action Steps

- *Stay realistic about the changes you can immediately expect to see now that he's taking T therapy; the Recovery Stage takes time.*
- *Make sure you understand the difference in attraction and libido. This will help you cope with your feelings of sexual rejection.*
- *Don't take it personally when he doesn't initiate; he has confidence-building work to do before he can get there.*
- *Don't worry about a lack of attraction and attachment at this point. You'll be rebuilding those as you move through each step in the Recovery Stage.*

# Chapter 16
# Healing the Injury
## *Step One*

In *Step One*, the main focus is going to be to reduce the negative interactions between the two of you. We're not going to add in positive interactions just yet; we're simply going to reduce the negative stuff that's slowing down your progress. These negative interactions are draining the life and energy out of both of you, making it impossible to heal.

You can think of this like that sports injury. After the injury is treated, what it most needs is time to heal. There is still a lot of pain and inflammation around the injured area. This is the body's way of protecting itself from further damage. People instinctively avoid putting pressure on the injured area during this stage because they know it will hurt!

The problem is that a breakdown in the three love systems is not visible to the naked eye in the same way a leg injury is. It's not as obvious that there is healing that needs to happen, and so in a low T marriage we don't instinctively know to avoid putting pressure on the 'injured area'.

In fact, over the last several years while your husband's hormones have been messed up, you've probably put a lot of pressure on him to be more sexual, to do more, to feel more, to talk to you more, and on and on. This is understandable. Your husband disappeared and you were trying to get him back. A certain amount of pressure was necessary to get him to make that doctor's appointment and address the problem. However, at this point in the recovery process, putting pressure on your husband to be more sexual and more attentive is actually going to be counter-productive and do more damage.

# Give It Time

At this point, you need to give your marriage time and space to heal. You want to avoid doing the things in your marriage that are actively causing damage. This is a frustrating stage because while your instinct is going to be to start doing active things to repair the marriage, what you really need to do at this point is to simply let it be. Take time to adjust to the new normal. Let your husband get used to being on testosterone therapy and give yourself time to adjust as well.

There is a huge mental shift for both the husband and wife when he gets a low T diagnosis; they stop thinking of him as indestructible and realize that his body isn't performing the way it used to. There's also a fair amount of grief that goes along with the realization. If you think back, you can see the stages of grief in both of your reactions; first denial, then disbelief, then anger and sadness. You both need time to process all of this.

# Have Realistic Expectations

For a long time, you've been starved for the sex and intimacy that you used to get from your marriage. It was natural for you to think that talking to your husband about the lack of them would help; however, by now you've figured out that talking about it really doesn't help at all. What you might not yet realize is that talking about it not only doesn't help, it actively hurts the recovery process. He can't perform the way you want him to right now; he's lost his conditioning.

Chances are that when your husband's sex drive first decreased, he was fairly neutral about having sex. It was as if his desire switch simply got shut off. It didn't bother him particularly because he didn't even notice it. When you're not hungry, you don't think about food one way or the other. However, as the months and years went by, you grew increasingly dissatisfied with the lack of sex and you started talking about it more and more.

While this is all completely natural and expected, it took your husband from being simply neutral about sex to actually feeling negative about it. This is also completely normal. If someone continually pressures you to have a Big Mac when you're not hungry, you eventually start feeling negative about going to McDonald's.

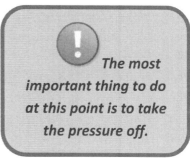

*The most important thing to do at this point is to take the pressure off.*

While low T was the original problem and your husband was initially neutral about having sex, he has probably developed a lot of negative feelings toward sex by this point and has become highly reactive to sexual expectations and pressure. He is likely feeling guilty about not wanting sex, emasculated by the fact that he doesn't, and resentful of the pressure you've put on him.

## Give Him Your Support

Picture that ballplayer who's been injured. He is sitting on the bench, watching the other players do what he used to love to do. His self-worth has taken a huge hit. Things that used to come easily to him seem to be out of his reach now. He wonders if he'll ever be as good as he used to be. This is the time when he most needs the support and encouragement of his teammates.

Now imagine how it would affect him if his teammates constantly criticized him for his lack of progress, if they expected more from him than his body was capable of, if they ignored his limp and expected him to get back into the game immediately. Can you picture how demoralizing this would be for him, and how it might impede his progress?

Yet this is what many women in a low T marriage do. Because your husband's injury isn't visible, you sometimes expect more from him than he can deliver. Knowing that he is disappointing you further demoralizes him.

You can't get what you want by treating him like the enemy. You simply can't. This is where I tell you to do hard things. You have to stop. You have to stop criticizing him about his missing sex drive; you have to stop yelling at him about it, you have to stop talking about sex *at all.* Trust me; I know how hard this is. I made all the same mistakes you're making, and I've watched other women do the same. You need to understand that you are substantially slowing down your progress by your actions.

## Stop the Death Spirals

Something else you need to do is to stop the Death Spirals. You know the drill … it's been a while since you had sex so you indicate to him in some manner that you're interested … and the clock starts  ticking. One night goes by with no initiation, you keep your cool. Then another night goes by and you start to get a tad bit testy. You become increasingly curt and irritated with him over the next couple of days; maybe you shut the cabinet doors a little harder than usual, maybe you give him the cool, silent treatment, maybe you start to criticize him for inconsequential things. The more you do these things, the more he withdraws. By the fourth night …. *There she blows!* You lose it. *What is* **wrong** *with him … the T therapy is supposed to give him a sex drive… he doesn't love you … he doesn't care …* All that pent up rage comes pouring out on his hapless head.

By the next day, you're embarrassed at your loss of control but in the moment, you simply lose it. While you never used to be so volatile, you've become hypersensitive to rejection.

> *Death Spirals happen when you feel sexually rejected by your husband and your anger grows out of control, causing further damage to the relationship.*

While it may temporarily feel better to indulge in a Death Spiral with him and he may even increase the sex frequency temporarily, in the long run it lowers his attraction for you and causes him to withdraw even further. While you can push him into having sex with you, you can't push him into feeling desire. You need to play the long game here.

So, no more temper tantrums about not getting sex. Let him heal. This is a confidence thing as much as it is a medical thing. You need to be his #1 fan. Anything you can do to increase his confidence is going to help him get back into the game more quickly.

## It Isn't Fair

You'll likely go through periods where you feel that it isn't fair that you have to do all this work just to get a normal sex life. And it isn't. But neither is breast cancer, famine, or childhood leukemia. Life isn't fair. I can't give you fairness, but I *can* tell you what will work the quickest to get the marriage you want.

It's going to take time for your husband to trust that the changes you're making are real and that you're not going to turn back into that critical shrew who complained all the time about the lack of sex.

He's also probably going to be oblivious to how bad you feel about being rejected. Hold your course. He's not malicious, he's just clueless as to the impact all of this has had on you. One day he'll get it, but not until he's had more time to recover. The longer he's been low T, the longer the recovery will be, so ... patience. You'll get there.

## Stop Being Needy

Think back to when you and your husband first started dating. There were a number of things that attracted him to you. You most likely had a lot going on in your life. You had friends, hobbies, and activities that you enjoyed. You were interesting and you were *fun*. You consistently showed high value by your words and by your actions. Your husband spent time with you because he wanted to, not because he felt obligated. He spent time with you because you were fun to be with.

Fast forward to the present. How have things changed with your dynamics? Do you still display value around your husband? Are you fun to be with or are your interactions marked by constant tension, criticism and arguments? Do you still do interesting things? Do you have a group of people you enjoy being with or are you frequently hanging around your husband in the hope that he'll want to spend time with you?

You have to stop showing low value by constantly circling your husband's feet like a little puppy begging for attention. I can't emphasize this enough. This is one of the main blockages to healing your marriage. You have to stop telling him that the two of you need to 'work on the marriage'. You have to stop crying because he'd rather play video games than spend time with you. The more you engage in these types of activities, the more damage it does to your marriage. The time is going to come when your husband looks forward to spending time with you again, but there's work to be done first.

## Set Reasonable Sexual Standards

When a man's testosterone levels first increase, there's an initial period where he starts feeling sexual again, but still lacks the energy

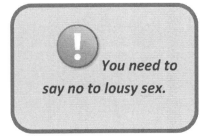
*You need to say no to lousy sex.*

and confidence to engage in good sex. You're so excited that he is actually showing desire again, and you're so used to taking whatever scraps he gives you, that you respond to him no matter how bad his initiation is. No time to connect first? *Fine*. Late at night when you're exhausted? *Fine*. A quickie in the morning when there's no time and you're waiting for the kids to walk in at any moment? *Fine*. No foreplay? *Fine*. The low T years have conditioned you to accept whatever he offers.

Again, I want you to think back to the days when you and your husband first started having sex together. Would you have accepted lousy sex back then? *Nope*. You valued yourself much more than that. So did he. You need to start showing value in this area again. You have to stop having crappy sex.

I know, you thought the whole point of fixing the low T was to get back to having sex. However, when you engage in sex that's easy for him but unsatisfying for you, it's a huge display of low value. What you're saying is that you aren't worth him putting in effort in order to have sex with you. When you have lousy sex with him, it lowers attraction for both of you.

In his mind, you having sex with him means that everything is fine. It sends him mixed signals. It's as if you put on a dress he hates but he tells you how great it looks on you, and then he wonders why you keep wearing it. I know that you think you're doing a good thing by having sex with him when he does some weak lazy bear initiation, but you're not. You really have to knock it off.

And yes, I know that means that you'll be getting even less sex than you do now, but you're playing the long game. The hot sex will come, but not quite yet. You have to delay gratification in order to get the results you want later. I'll expand on this in Chapter 19, but for now, just know that it's okay to set reasonable boundaries when it comes to sex.

## Track Marital Satisfaction

Something else that's useful at this point is to start tracking your marital satisfaction on a scale of 1-100. It's going to be low right now, but I want you to have a baseline against which to compare. There are going to be times in the upcoming weeks when you feel like the two of you are making no progress at all and you're going to get discouraged. I want you to be able to see that your marriage is gradually improving as you eliminate some of the negative interactions we discussed in this chapter. It won't be a linear process, there will be peaks and valleys, but over time, you'll see a gradual upward progression in your marital satisfaction.

# What to Expect at this Point

- *This is probably the most frustrating step of the Recovery Stage because some of the repairs you're making aren't visible and progress will seem slow. Hang in there.*
- *You'll experience a rollercoaster as your husband see-saws between his old self and the new normal.*
- *It will be difficult to avoid falling into old patterns of criticism and negative emotion.*
- *You may wonder if he's even trying and will probably feel angry at him for not trying harder. Give him time, he's going to get there.*

# Action Steps

- *Reduce the pressure you put on him and give him time and space to adjust and heal.*
- *Be as encouraging and supportive as possible.*
- *Set reasonable standards for sex.*
- *Track marital satisfaction on a scale of 1-100.*

That's it. I know it's easier said than done, but all of this effort will eventually pay off. As you gradually engage in these new behaviors, you'll see the positive energy in your marriage grow. This will lay the groundwork for the next step of the *Recovery Stage*.

# Chapter 17
# Cleared for Practice
## *Step Two*

If you've done the things in *Step One* to reduce your negative interactions, you should be seeing less conflict in your marriage at this point. You're probably finding that you and your husband are arguing less and things are less volatile. Good work on reducing those negative interactions! I know how tough it is.

Decreasing the negative interactions in *Step One* reduced the drain on both of you and will allow the two of you to focus on the main goal of *Step Two;* increasing your personal energy and attractiveness.

This is a necessary next step because while the reduced conflict has improved attachment, it hasn't done much for attraction. It's true that things are more peaceful and you feel more comfortable with each other, but it's probably left somewhat of a void. At least when the two of you were fighting all the time, he was noticing you.

At this point, you feel more invisible to him than ever! Sex is no better, either. You're still acting like roommates, and you're wondering, "Now what? Is this how it's going to be? Where do we go from here?" Don't give up hope because you're going to start changing all of that by increasing personal energy and attractiveness.

## Train Separately

You'll do this by focusing on yourself rather than on your husband, or even on the marriage. That may seem counter-intuitive, but it makes sense when you realize that the low testosterone years didn't just affect your husband, they affected you as well.

Your energy and confidence have taken a hit just as his have, and you have some repair work to do just as he does. In a sense, *both* of you are cleared for practice and you *both* need to get out there and strengthen yourselves in order to get back into the game.

## Increase Energy

A woman in a low T marriage tends to spend so much mental energy thinking about what is going on with her husband that she neglects her own life. She becomes hyper-focused on him, and stops doing the things that enrich her life.

High energy is attractive. Positivity is attractive. People who do interesting things are attractive. Chances are that your energy and positivity have decreased during your husband's low T years.

Why is this? Well, energy is also contagious. As your husband became less energetic and more fatigued, it affected not only his own energy, but also yours. Then as your positive

> **High energy and positivity are attractive.**

energy decreased, it impacted your husband. The two of you got into a vicious cycle where you each pulled the other's energy down. That part needs to change.

In this chapter, we'll focus on doing the things that increase your own personal energy and the attraction in your marriage. They fall into two basic categories, *physical* and *internal frame*, as summarized in Table 13.

Making physical changes in your life is vital to increasing your energy. Getting to the gym, dressing better, going out and doing fun things, these are all great ways to gain the energy that makes you more attractive.

It's important, though, to work on your internal frame as well, something people often neglect. Internal frame refers to the emotional/psychological components of increasing energy. The value you place on yourself determines the way other people see you. Confidence, being generally fun to be around, and setting reasonable boundaries all increase your own personal value and energy.

| Ways to Increase Positive Energy and Attraction | |
|---|---|
| **Physical** | **Internal Frame** |
| • Get out and do stuff. | • Regain your confidence. |
| • Work on your girl game. | • Show high value. |
| • Make a dating profile. | • Increase your date-ability quotient. |
| • Make lifestyle changes. | • Set reasonable boundaries. |
| | • Understand that anger is unattractive and unproductive. |
| | • Get rid of the 'Good Girl'. |
| | • Stop accepting 'peace at any price'. |

Table 13

# Physical - Get Out and Do Stuff

You need to stop looking to your husband to supply energy, he simply doesn't have enough to spare at this point. That will eventually change, but not yet. Instead, you need to start doing the activities that bring energy and flow into your own life. What are those things you used to love doing when you were single? Start doing those again. It doesn't much matter what. Just start adding small things into your life that make you feel more positive and energetic.

Here are some examples of ways that various women increased their energy:

- *One woman rediscovered her passion for photography and started entering and winning photo contests. She is turning it into a second career.*
- *Another woman remembered how much she enjoyed snowshoeing and started participating in the sport again.*
- *One woman reignited her career by finishing a training manual she had been working on for years.*

- *Another completed a certification she needed to take her career to the next level.*
- *Another woman resumed a side career she loved but had let lapse.*

All of these things increased each woman's positivity and energy. But you don't necessarily have to do big things. Even small things will increase your energy. Here are some examples to inspire you:

- *Challenge yourself to get strong enough to do a pull-up.*
- *Clean out a closet that's been driving you nuts.*
- *Redecorate a room that's outlived its original purpose.*
- *Plant a container garden.*
- *Learn a new sport.*
- *Volunteer at the public library.*
- *Find a new hiking group.*
- *Organize all your pics into digital scrapbooks.*

It can really be just about anything. Anything that excites and inspires you, anything that brings you flow. Stop making excuses not to do it. Stop waiting for your husband to get on-board. What would you do if your husband disappeared tomorrow? Go do those things now.

Getting out there in the wide wide world, trying new activities, accomplishing new goals, and having fun all lead to the next step.

## Internal Frame - Regain Your Confidence

As your husband's T levels dropped and his sexual desire diminished, you thought there was something wrong with you and your confidence took a hit. Even though you now know that this simply wasn't the case, it's going to take some work to change those neural pathways in your brain and restore the confidence and vibrancy you used to have.

As you start tackling the challenges in this section one by one, you will find that you view yourself differently. One of the most effective ways to change the way you see yourself is to work on your girl game.

# Physical - Work on Your Girl Game

In a marriage where both partners are healthy and functional, they are normally responsive to each other; that is, when one person starts upping their game substantially - losing weight, working out, dressing better, etc. - the other partner usually follows behind.

The reverse is also true. When your husband's T levels decreased, he lost energy and dropped his game. For a while, you tried to get him to gain energy by working out, losing weight, doing fun things, etc., but after a while you simply gave up. At that point you probably also dropped your own game a bit. After all, what's the point of trying to attract a husband who never even seems to notice you? It felt pointless to keep trying to attract him during the low T fog. But all of that is changing now that his hormones are back to optimal. Now is the time to re-focus on your girl game.

There's nothing like working on your girl game to increase personal energy in your life. What is girl game, exactly? Girl game is all the stuff that acts on a man's dopamine centers and makes a woman attractive to him. It encompasses her figure, her make-up, her hair, her wardrobe, her sexuality and her sense of being fun and flirty. Many women submerge their sexuality when their husband's energy decreases due to low T. You need to bring that stuff out of hiding, but how? Take a look at the 'Girl Game' box on the next page for ideas.

It's important to realize that you're making these changes *for you*. Don't look to your husband for affirmation of what you're working on; at this point, his response will likely only disappoint you. You've lived the last several years gauging your value based on his response to you; it's time to break that pattern.

The hotter you are in a relationship, the more leverage you have with your partner. As your husband sees you getting more and more attractive, he will intuitively understand that you have options and this will increase his motivation to make the changes he needs to make.

## Girl Game

***Get to the Gym*** - The first thing you need to do is to get to the gym. I can hear you groaning, but you need to develop the confidence and energy that come from working out. Get a personal trainer if you need to in order to set goals and get accountability.

***New Wardrobe*** - If you still have stuff in your closet from ten years ago, get ruthless and start clearing it out. Stop dressing like a nun and wear clothes that emphasize your femininity. You don't want to look like a tramp, but stop wearing things that are two sizes too large. If your budget is tight, try consignment stores. You can find great buys there.

***New Hair and Make-Up*** - Same thing with your hair and make-up. If you haven't changed them since you were in high school, now's the time. Get a professional consultation or take a look at YouTube; there are a million how-to videos there.

***Fun and Flirty*** - For most of us, this is the hardest part. We haven't flirted with our husband in ages and we've forgotten how to do it. You need to start practicing. Flirting is simply a matter of showing interest in and being friendly to other people, and you can do that with almost anyone; grandmas and grandpas, young kids, other women, etc. Start practicing eye contact and having conversations with other people you meet during the day. Smile at people you pass. If you don't get out during the day enough to flirt, then go back and take another look at *'Get Out and Do Stuff'*.

***Build Healthy Friendships*** - This is a key point in your improvements. Surround yourself with a group of people who are healthy, fun and functional. You need to have options apart from your husband. It's as true now as it was when you were single.

# Physical - Make a Dating Profile

Now that you're working on your girl game, make a dating profile just for kicks. Don't post it on a dating website though, no matter how much you're tempted! This exercise is simply to let you see yourself as others might see you. Are you doing interesting things? Have you made the most of your appearance? Are you a fun person to be around? Are you attractive to the opposite sex? What are the areas in your life that need the most work?

If you can't fill out the fun sections of a dating profile, then you have to face the fact that you've become boring! This becomes your starting point. Go back to the *'Get Out and Do Stuff'* section and figure out what fun and interesting things you are going to do first.

While making a dating profile falls under physical improvements, there is also a huge internal frame component to it as well. Looking at yourself from an outside perspective helps you see areas where your internal frame is weak and needs work.

# Internal Frame - Show High Value

For a long time now, you've displayed low value to your husband. You've accepted a less than satisfying sex life, you've complained about it, but never taken action, you've been angry and critical; you've been low energy and possibly boring. You've continually pursued him and wanted more from him than he was able to give. You've told him by your actions that you'll accept anything he hands out to you. You've put a low value on your own worth and your husband accepted your valuation.

You need to start showing high value. What does that look like exactly? When you show high value, you don't wait for someone to rescue you; Prince Charming is not on his way. You don't wait around for your husband to provide all your dopamine and your stimulation. Remember what your mom used to tell you? Boring people are bored ... and bored people are boring. It's just as true now that you're married as it was back then. You have to make your own excitement and provide your own stimulation.

Women tend to be responsive to men, wanting our husbands to be the leaders in our home. That will come, but not yet. For now, you can't sit around waiting for your husband to take the lead because he's not quite ready.

Stop waiting for him to plan a Date Night; instead, come up with a plan of your own. "Honey, I'm going out for Mexican. Do you want to come?" If he doesn't, it's no biggie because you have several girlfriends who would love to go. Because you're a fun and interesting person. Do you see how this works? You *want* his company, but you don't *need* it because you're a person of high value who is quite capable of attracting friends who want to do things with you. You have options; he is only one of many.

## Internal Frame - Increase Your Date-ability Quotient

Along the same lines, are you date-able? Take a minute to think about the behaviors you exhibit with your husband. If you acted the same way with a new guy, would he ask you out on a date? Your husband was first attracted to you because you were fun to be with. Are you still fun when you're with him? Or is that reserved only for friends and co-workers?

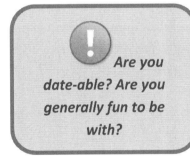

*Are you date-able? Are you generally fun to be with?*

In order to be date-able, you need to be generally pleasant and positive. You need to be interested and interesting. You need to find something to talk about other than the kids or the latest house repairs. You need to look your best, whatever that best may be.

What does this look like in action? It might be more productive to show what it *doesn't* look like. Let's take a look at Jack and Diane, who are trying to get their marriage back on track after many low T years.

## A Little Ditty About Jack and Diane

*Jack asks Diane out on a date. He hints that maybe they should have sex when they get home since it's been a while. Diane is unenthusiastic about going out with him because his dates are usually pretty boring, to be honest. He always wants to go out to eat, which is her least favorite thing to do. He also never plans ahead, so things frequently fall through the cracks. This has been the source of many an argument between the two of them.*

*Sure enough, Jack makes plans to go to a local restaurant. Diane sighs and rolls her eyes. In the hours prior to the date, Diane frantically tries to get the house clean before the sitter gets there, growing increasingly resentful that Jack isn't helping.*

*When it's time to leave, Diane still hasn't had time to do her hair or make-up, so she pulls her hair back into a ponytail and throws on some jeans. His fault, she thinks, for not helping her get things done around the house.*

*By the time they get to the restaurant, Diane is fuming and Jack is increasingly withdrawn, fearing the rage volcano pouring down on his head. When Diane opens her menu to discover that there are no vegetarian choices available, she really lets him have it! He's a poor planner, he doesn't care about her or whether she has anything she can eat, he never helps out, and he's boring.*

*They drive home in stiff silence. Once home, Jack immediately disappears downstairs. As the hour grows later, Diane realizes that he's not going to initiate yet again, and she goes to bed furious and hurt. The T therapy hasn't helped at all!*

This scenario may sound exaggerated, but it's based on numerous interactions I've seen in recovering low T couples. Do you recognize yourself in any of it? Diane's on-going resentment with Jack poisons most of their interactions. She's never going to get the positive outcome she wants until she starts acting positively. If she acted this way with a stranger, she wouldn't be asked out for a second date. She's failed the date-ability test.

## Internal Frame - Set Reasonable Boundaries

Don't confuse 'acting pleasant and positive' with being a doormat. I'm not telling you to 'play nice', and accept anything your husband offers. In fact, just the opposite. People who show high value have strong boundaries. They know what they're willing to accept or not accept. They're not angry all the time because they don't allow their boundaries to be continually trampled.

Again, let's take a look at that in action. What would have happened if Diane had told Jack that while she wanted to go out with him, she'd like to go roller-skating after dinner? The energy would have been immediately higher for both of them. What if she had done some research and found a few restaurants that had vegetarian choices and asked Jack to choose one of them? What if she had asked Jack to help her clean the house instead of playing the martyr role and trying to get it all done on her own?

Do you see what happened? Diane didn't set appropriate boundaries with Jack, and that made a positive outcome impossible. She was content to remain in the victim role and until she stops doing that, her marriage is not going to progress. Boundaries are attractive, anger isn't.

## Hey, You Tricked Me!

My guess is that this is the part of the book where you start to feel angry. I pulled somewhat of a bait and switch on you. I told you that the book was going to fix your husband's low testosterone, but I didn't say anything about you having to make changes. However, the truth is that if you don't make changes, you will never have the marriage you want. And the most important change you have to make is to get past the anger that is poisoning every interaction between you and your husband.

# Internal Frame - Understand that Anger is Unattractive

If there's one thing that women in low T marriages share (other than a lack of sex, that is), it's *anger.* We are all furious. We're angry with the husbands who rejected us ... at the medical system that failed us ... at our sex-less lives ... at *ourselves* for putting up with an intolerable situation for so long.

This anger is part of the low T script and while it's normal to feel it, it's getting in the way of having the marriage you want. What you may not realize is how unattractive your anger is to your husband. As long as you are angry with him, you are diminishing his ability to be attracted to you and his desire to connect with you.

It started out that low T was the problem in the marriage, but at this point your anger is poisoning the marriage every bit as much as the original low T. The bitterness you've felt has changed you. Each time you are angry and critical with him over every little thing, it diminishes attraction and he simply shuts down.

You've grown comfortable with your victim role, and the pain of being rejected has started feeling *normal,* but being a victim won't get your marriage back on track. Only positive action can do that.

# Internal Frame - Understand that Anger is Unproductive

As well as being unattractive, anger is also unproductive. Anger is a good tool for recognizing when someone is trampling all over your boundaries, but it's a lousy tool for bringing about positive change. So how do you get past feeling so bitterly angry over the years you've lost to low T?

Earlier in the book, I briefly mentioned that the reason you feel so angry is that you feel powerless. All these years, you have felt powerless to get the marriage and sex life you want. No matter what you did or how hard you tried, nothing seemed to change in your marriage. However you actually had the power to change things all along, you just didn't realize it.

For a long time, you've been blaming your husband for the problems in your marriage. You are so used to seeing him as the bad guy that you can't see how you contributed to the problems. Yes, he wasn't willing to look for solutions with you and was content to hide his head in the sand for far too long. But you need to realize that your husband couldn't have acted the way he did if you had not accepted it. You did a lot of talking about the problem and you did a lot of complaining about the problem, but you never took action that said, "Hey, this is unacceptable. I won't live like this."

# Internal Frame - Get Rid of that 'Good Girl'

This is very common 'good girl' behavior. Good girls tend to be people pleasers, conditioned to put others' needs ahead of their own. When they do this, they get lost in the shuffle and their resentment grows while they wait for someone else to recognize and meet their needs. Good girls don't want to be seen as selfish or self-centered.

Good girls are also afraid of conflict. They don't like to make waves by making demands and therefore they never get their own needs met. The good girl in you is what kept you from setting reasonable boundaries about your husband's low testosterone for so long and allowed your marriage to become so dysfunctional. You've got to get rid of that girl, she's no good for you!

# Internal Frame - Stop Accepting Peace at Any Price

"When you believe in peace at any price, the price of peace gets higher and higher." When I first read those words, a lightbulb went off in my head. It helped me understand that the reason my husband had walked all over me was because I hadn't set good boundaries, and the reason I was angry was because I felt powerless to change my situation.

This was not my husband's fault. He hadn't taken my power away from me, I had handed it over to him. Giftwrapped it, in fact!

Until you accept responsibility for the part you played in the problems in your marriage, you will handicap your progress. To be quite honest, I was very slow in getting to this realization. I hung onto the anger and victimhood for far too long and it really slowed

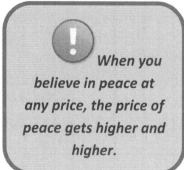

*When you believe in peace at any price, the price of peace gets higher and higher.*

our progress down. I'd like to help you avoid that if possible.

# Internal Frame - Take Power and Set Boundaries

You have to make changes in your life so that you can stop being angry. You keep thinking that if only your husband would change, you could stop being angry. It's counter-intuitive, but letting go of the anger has nothing at all to do with your husband, and everything to do with you.

That's why the actions in *Step Two* all focus on you. You have to take power over your own life in order to stop feeling angry. Once you start doing the things that bring you flowing energy, your husband's actions will no longer control your emotions. When you fill your life up with the things that bring you joy, your anger will dissipate.

> *Being angry = Not having power*
> *Having power = Not being angry*

As you follow the suggestions in *Step Two* and make the changes that increase your own personal energy and attractiveness, you will find that you stop being so dependent on your husband for your happiness.

In fact, you will probably find that your husband starts orbiting *you* as he finds you growing increasingly happy and independent. This is a necessary step to right the dynamics in your marriage that had become so dysfunctional in the low T years.

## Make Lifestyle Changes

There are a ton of tools for you in this chapter. You're trying to change ingrained behaviors, and just like your husband has to change his neural pathways, so do you. It's time to start incorporating the lifestyle changes that help you change the way your brain is wired. You don't have to do them all at once; just gradually add them into your life. They will help you make the internal frame changes you need to make in order move to the next level.

| Lifestyle Changes that Promote New Neural Pathways |
|---|
| • Continue Working Out |
| • Eat Healthier |
| • Get Some Sunshine |
| • Do Something Creative |
| • Develop a New Hobby |
| • Reduce stress |
| • Get Better Sleep |

Table 14

# What to Expect at this Point

- *This step of the Recovery Stage involves a lot of hard work, but the payoff is huge.*
- *You will find that your energy increases as you make some of the changes in this chapter, and you're going to start having fun. You'll find a whole big world out there.*
- *You will feel years younger.*

- *Your confidence will increase.*
- *You will gain a gradually growing sense of peace as you recognize that your husband is not your only vendor; you are a woman with options.*
- *You may feel a growing sense of distance from your husband. That's okay, it's a result of looking inward rather than outward, and it's a necessary step in the process.*
- *Your husband will start to value you more; so will the other people in your life.*
- *You will start getting more attention from other people, particularly men.*

# Action Steps

- *Increase your energy and build an interesting life.*
- *Increase your date-ability quotient.*
- *Work on your girl game.*
- *When you feel yourself growing angry with your husband, take a step back and analyze whether your anger over a specific incident is reasonable or whether it's generalized anger from years of negative interactions between the two of you.*
- *Set strong boundaries.*
- *Include lifestyle changes that support your new growth. Pick two options per month from the 'Life Style Changes' in Table 14 until you've incorporated them all.*

# Chapter 18
# Getting Back in the Game
*Step Three*

The two of you have made a lot of progress. You've reduced the negative interactions that were piling on more damage to the marriage and increased your own personal energy and attractiveness.

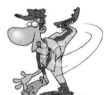

Up until now, we've focused on strengthening each of you as individuals rather than concentrating on your interactions together. By this point, however, you're finally ready to start playing together as a team. This is going to involve consciously and intentionally engaging in teamwork, and adding the activities and routines that build both attraction and attachment.

In *Step Three*, we're going to focus on five different areas. This may sound like a lot, but I think you'll find that you've built a strong enough foundation in *Steps One* and *Two* to be able to handle *Step Three*.

- *Work together*
- *Play together*
- *Remember to be lovers*
- *Do the things that attract each other*
- *Celebrate your successes together*

## Work Together

One common dynamic in a low T marriage is that as a man's energy levels decrease, he becomes increasingly disconnected from his wife and family. He loses his confidence and ability to make decisions. Decisions and leadership fall more and more to his wife, whether she wants it or not, and they stop working together as a couple. This shift in dynamics affects both the wife's respect for her husband as well as his respect for himself. This decreases attraction for both of them and lessens their feelings of attachment. Both the dopamine and oxytocin love systems are impacted.

If you are experiencing this dynamic in your marriage, you may feel a bit like a single mom, struggling to handle all the decisions on your own. This is a common pattern in a marriage where the guy has had low T for a long time. In *Step Three*, we're going to work on changing all that. While you may be at a loss as to how to change your dynamics, there are tools that can help.

## Set Common Goals

It's typical in a long-term, low T marriage for a couple to stop setting goals together. As the husband's energy and motivation wane, and the wife's anger and resentment build, they simply stop working together as a team. You may have found that you and your husband have been drifting for a while, having only enough energy to manage the most basic day-to-day functions. Now that the energy level in your marriage is rising, it's time to start planning together again.

## Bring Him into the Loop

You need to pull your husband back into the loop regarding family matters. Take a look at the things you handle for the family. Maybe that's the insurance, the banking, and the kids' school stuff. Take an evening each week and work together to bring your husband up to speed in each area. Write down websites and passwords you use, the kids' teachers' names, their daily schedule, etc. Your husband can't make intelligent decisions if he doesn't have the information he needs.

## Have Weekly Planning Meetings

One tool that works well for bringing him into the loop is weekly planning meetings. Start setting aside a specific time each week to sit down and talk about your goals. You can start small, simply discussing the week's activities and schedule, and what needs to get accomplished for that particular week. Over time, the goal is to build up to covering long-term goals for your marriage, finances, family, and careers.

# Shifting Leadership - How Did It Get So Bad?

Like many men in the low T fog, when my husband's T levels were low, he was simply worn out, and I increasingly tried to spare him from dealing with problems. Broken windows and appliances that were making funny noises. Kids' misbehavior and financial woes. School open houses and after-school activities. I tried to handle all of those things because he was so overwhelmed and exhausted all the time. The kids learned not to bother their dad with problems, and increasingly came to me for each decision. We weren't working together anymore, and with five kids, the stress was taking a toll on my energy.

Those were dark years for him, and he struggled simply to keep things on track at work. In an effort to support him, I took on more and more on the domestic front. I simply made decisions and moved on. By the time we saw each other in the evenings, we were both out of energy and communication was minimal. Plus, there was so much anger and resentment between us over our sexual dysfunction that there were many nights we didn't talk at all, we just retreated to our separate corners.

Our dynamics had become really dysfunctional! The way we had done things during the low T years had been necessary to a certain extent but once my husband addressed the low T, we needed to make changes in the way we handled decisions and leadership. Once his T levels were optimal, my husband was full of energy and completely capable of taking charge and making decisions. I came to the realization that if I wanted him to take a leadership role in our family, I had to do my part and provide him with the tools to do so. One tool was information. I needed to make sure that he had access to the same information about the kids that I did. This meant that we needed an intentional way to communicate rather than sporadically sharing dribs and drabs of information.

A baseball coach regularly meets with his players not only to provide information, but also to give a vision for where the team needs to go and how they're going to get there. It's the same with your planning meeting. You and your husband need to set priorities for your marriage and family, and get on the same page about how to reach your goals.

This has been one of the most important things my husband and I have done to build our marriage. When we first started, we were just leaving the low T fog behind and our marriage was still dysfunctional. The weekly planning meetings were distinctly ... *chilly*. We kept them brisk and business-like, discussing various kids' activities, who was taking whom where, and what projects needed to get done around the house that week.

They gradually grew to encompass conversations about our personal goals, our goals for our kids and our careers, and our long term vision for where we wanted to be in five ... ten ... fifteen years. We now look forward to having that time together to reconnect each week, bringing our coffee with us and settling in comfortably to discuss what's going on in our world.

I've learned some tips along the way, both from my own marriage, and also from coaching other couples. On the next page you'll find suggestions for making your weekly planning meetings as productive as possible.

## *Hold Family Meetings*

An adjunct to this is to have a family meeting once a week as well. This is a quick meeting where you look at the weekly schedule and make sure everyone knows what's going on for the week.

You can use it to discuss each kid's extra-curricular activities for the week and who is taking whom where. Discuss the chores that need to get done around the house and any problems that have come up during the week. Keep it short. Again, you don't want to get weighed down with these tools. 15-20 minutes should do it and everyone goes away feeling more connected.

# Tips for Weekly Planning Meetings

*Keep the same time each week* as much as possible. You want to get in the habit of doing these meetings; otherwise, they'll fall by the wayside. When you're insanely busy is the time you most need to have your meeting so the two of you can stay on the same page.

*Pick a time where you won't get interrupted.* For us, this is Sunday afternoons. We're more relaxed and not so tired from work. If your kids are younger, park them in front of a movie or other entertainment to buy yourself some time. Turn off your phones, shut the door and make this a priority.

*Keep it simple* at first. There's no need to get too ambitious all at once. Start by looking at your weekly schedule and the kids' activities. After a while, maybe throw in meal planning for the week. At some point, you'll want to develop a budget together. Eventually, it will become more of a vision meeting and less of a planning meeting, but you want to let it all flow organically and not get bogged down with planning too much at once.

*Avoid talking about relationship problems* during this meeting. Keep it positive and productive. Relationship talks can become a quagmire. Save the heavy relationship discussions for later.

*Keep track of the discussion.* What works for us is to put the notes straight into our laptop or phone and send the other one a copy. Whatever works for you is fine. You just need some way of tracking what your goals are. Post them somewhere and mark them off as they get done.

*Follow up* each week to see what got done and what didn't. We've become competitive about our goals, trying to out-do each other. We're usually scrambling toward the end of the week to fit it all in, but the competition makes it more fun and keeps our energy levels high. Play around with it and see what works best for you.

Now that you've established your family meetings, it's time to take it a step further. If you want your husband to take a leadership role with the kids, he needs to know what's going on in their lives. Set aside time each week to talk to each kid individually. Keep the meetings short, the goal is to increase positive energy, not to get bogged down with a cumbersome duty. You're just quickly touching base on what's going on in each kid's life, how they are feeling, and anything they need to share.

Eventually, these meetings can go a bit deeper. We've gotten great results from having our kids rate their life satisfaction on a scale from 1-10. Anything under a 7 becomes a red flag that something needs to change. It's kind of an early warning detection system.

This more than anything else is going to help your husband get back in touch with his family. It has been heart-warming to see my husband re-connect with our kids. Recently, for example, my husband had to run to the hardware store for some supplies. Our college-aged son decided to go with him. When my husband asked if our son needed anything, our son replied, "No, I just want to spend some time with you, Dad." Five years ago, that never would have happened. Changes are possible. You just need the tools to make them happen.

### *Give Him Room to Lead*

One caveat is that you will probably be tempted to take over during these meetings, both with the individual child and during the family meeting. After all, you've been in charge for a while, and you're not quite sure if your husband can manage all this. He can. He won't do it quite like you do, but that's okay. He'll eventually find his footing and his own style of managing the family. Give him the time and space to do so. You really will reap tremendous rewards.

## Play Together

A common problem in marriages, particularly in low T marriages, is that a couple stops playing together and having fun with each other. Think back to when you were first attracted to each other. Chances are that the vast majority of your interactions involved fun, engaging experiences together. This is crucial to building attraction between two people. Research tells us that when people engage in high intensity, exciting activities together, they become more attracted to each other. In fact, the more adrenaline produced from an activity, the higher the feelings of attraction. In order to repair the dopamine love system in your marriage, you need to start doing the things that increase your attraction for each other. There are a million different ways you can do this.

## Go Out on Dopamine Dates

Take another look at your regular date nights. My guess is that if you go out on dates at all, they probably involve going out to dinner, with maybe an occasional stop at the hardware store to pick up the supplies you need for your next project. On rare occasions, maybe you

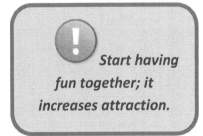

**Start having fun together; it increases attraction.**

throw in a movie. *Woo Hoo*! I see you smiling out there because you know I'm right. But here's the thing, all of that is *boring*. There's no excitement in any of that, no adrenaline, no dopamine. Your 22-year-old self would be horrified at the life you're

currently living. Boring people are *bored* ... and the two of you are bored with each other. So, time to change all that.

What you want to do is to add in some dopamine date nights. It's not all that difficult. I've worked with people who have done dance lessons, rock climbing, ropes courses, trampoline bounce houses, hiking, visiting new places, etc. The list really is endless. You simply have to think outside the box. When the two of you engage in these types of activities together, you will find that you become more attractive to each other. Remember, high energy is attractive. Fun is attractive. When we do high energy, fun things, we draw people to us. It's just as true now as it was when you were 20.

Here's a list just to get you started. Try planning one high energy date night per month and see how it goes. Just one to start with. My guess is that you're going to get hooked once you see the difference it makes in your interactions together. We know from multiple studies that couples who participate together in exciting, intense activities report more satisfaction with the relationship and feeling more 'in love' with each other. Give it a shot and see how it works.

---

# Ideas for Dopamine Dates

- *Hiking*
- *Paintball*
- *Laser tag*
- *Salsa or other types of dancing*
- *Ropes courses*

- *Trampoline bounce houses*
- *Exploring new places*
- *Geocaching*
- *Wine tastings*
- *Ice skating or roller skating*

---

## Incorporate Dopamine Moments

Of course, the problem with dopamine date nights is that they're not all that frequent. That's why you also need to incorporate some fun during the week. I've seen couples get great results from doing this. It doesn't have to be huge or time-consuming. Start small. Put a beanbag game out on your back deck. Challenge your husband to a game; it takes ten minutes. Up the ante by having the loser pay a forfeit. Maybe he has to go get ice cream for the two of you. Put up a dartboard in your garage. Play a game or two after dinner. Don't overthink it. Just steal little moments here and there.

One couple I worked with had a great time playing hide 'n seek in the dark after the kids were in bed. One couple got a huge kick out of having surprise squirt-gun fights. Buy some Nerf guns and have a shoot-out. It can be as simple as a quick game of poker, played with forfeits. As attraction grows, the forfeits become more extreme. Shoot some hoops. If you have a Wii, play the sword fight game where you knock each other off cliffs. My husband and I love that one, and it usually leads to some wrestling and general horseplay. Thumb wrestle or wrestle around on the bed together. Challenge him to arm-wrestle you. Anything that's active and competitive will work. Anything that gets you laughing and sweaty and out of breath. All of that builds attraction.

Here's your next assignment. Plan two small dopamine moments for next week. Again, you're going to start small so that you don't feel overwhelmed. Eventually, you'll add more and they'll become more spontaneous. After a couple of weeks of doing this, see whether the energy and attraction in your marriage has grown. My guess is that you'll see significant improvements. Give it a try and see what happens.

## *Work Out Together*

As part of your general efforts to become more attractive, you've each started working out. You can ratchet that up a notch by working out together. This provides double benefits because you get more attractive at the same time that you build attraction by being active together. This works well for a lot of couples.

If you can't manage to exercise at the same time, try doing the same workout at different times. Because of our schedules, my husband and I can't get to the gym together, but we use the same gym and do the same workout even though it's at different times. We've become quite competitive about it and try to out-do each other with our progress. My husband teases me unmercifully about being such a weakling and I do the same thing to him about his lack of flexibility. These are all little points of interaction that create connection and attraction.

You can also try new sports together. Join a co-ed league or take fencing lessons together. Hike together or try out a new martial art together. Learn to ski. Take snorkeling lessons. Again, there's really no limit. We live in a world where there are hundreds of activities and lessons on offer; you simply have to make the first move. The beauty of it is that all of these physical activities will increase testosterone … for both of you. This means that you're working on all three love systems at once. Time spent together increases your attachment bond; intense adrenaline activity increases your attraction for each other, and physical exertion increases testosterone, which improves your general hormone system. It's a win-win-win.

### Provide Your Own Dopamine

One common mistake wives in low T marriages make is that they rely exclusively on their husband to provide the dopamine. They basically sit back and say, "Attract me." This doesn't work, especially if you're the higher stimulation partner. While it's true that women are highly reactive to a man's energy and it's normal to want your husband to be a strong leader in your marriage, you have to give him something to work with. Don't be afraid to start the ball rolling by planning the first few activities.

As you add more dopamine into your relationship, you're going to find that the momentum in your relationship improves, making it easier for your husband to keep the ball rolling. Be forgiving of the occasional activity that turns out to be a bust. This is all simply playing together to see what works for the two of you. Build off each other and tweak it as often as needed until you find a good mix.

## Remember to be Lovers

It's so important in any marriage to remember that you're not just partners, you're not just parents, you're not just teammates, you're also lovers. That's what you were before any of the rest, and it's the heart of your union. It's especially important in a low T marriage because when your husband's libido decreased, so did his sense of being your

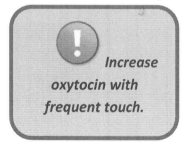

*Increase oxytocin with frequent touch.*

lover. It takes practice for him to rebuild those neural pathways. Lots and lots of practice.

### Touch Base When You First Get Home

One way to remember that you're lovers is to structure your so that you have time to reconnect when you first get home from work. Take five or ten minutes, however much you can manage, to go in your bedroom and shut the world outside your door. Then lie on the bed and touch or hold each other. You don't even need to talk, in fact, it's better if you don't talk. Look into each other's eyes, hold hands, put your head on his shoulder, let him stroke your hair, whatever. Just take time to reconnect in a physical way.

Remember that when you touch each other, your body produces the bonding and trust hormone, oxytocin. Oxytocin reinforces your pair bond and increases feelings of attachment. If you can only manage five minutes before the kids come pounding on your door, that's fine. Try this for the next few weeks and see how it works for you. I think you'll find that your attachment bond grows stronger.

## Reconnect Before Bed

Take some time to be together again in the evening simply to touch and be touched. This is the time to get more sensual. The kids are in bed, the house is quiet, and the two of you are winding down. Unplug from screen time for at least half an hour before bed. Light some candles in your bedroom and lie down together and touch. Run a bath and bathe together. Give each other a massage. Make it slow and sensual. Put some of your favorite lingerie on and let your husband take it off. If it leads to sex, that's great. But if not, you are strengthening your oxytocin bond with each touch. This is an important part of the low T recovery process, simply getting to know each other's bodies again and building your feelings of attachment.

Give it a whirl this week and see how it goes. You can start small, maybe two evenings each week. Gradually increase until you're up to at least four or five evenings each week. You'll find yourself looking forward to it each day, and eventually your day will seem incomplete until you have that time together.

# Do the Things that Attract Each Other

This one seems remarkably obvious, but it's surprising how many people simply miss it. Each of us has attraction triggers. Whether it's dangly earrings on a woman, or a pair of work boots on a guy, we're attracted to specific things. Attraction isn't a choice. You can love someone (oxytocin love system) without being attracted to them (dopamine love system).

Now, if I were writing this book for guys, I would focus on what he could do to attract you, but he's not here, you are! That means we're going to focus on the things you can do to attract him. However, there *are* some great resources in the back of the book to help your husband build attraction in the marriage.

## Do the Things that Attract Him

For my husband, it's long hair and skirts. The guy loves when I wear my hair long and I wear skirts. It's kind of embarrassing to admit, but for years I pretty much ignored this fact. I vaguely knew that he liked my hair when it was longer, but I didn't realize how important it was to him. Likewise with skirts. For years, I stopped wearing skirts. No particular reason why. Just didn't. It wasn't until we actively started working to build attraction that I had the 'aha'

> **If you want your husband to find you attractive, you need to do the things that attract him.**

moment. "Wow, if I want my husband to be attracted to me, I need to do the things he finds attractive."

Now that I wear my hair longer, I can't count the times he runs his hands through it and tells me how beautiful it is. Or the times where I'll catch him staring at me, and say, "What?" and he'll say, "Your hair looks so shiny in that light." Or the way his eyes light up when he walks in the door to find me in a skirt. And how he can't stop himself from running his hand up my leg. How could I have missed this for so long?

If you want your husband to find you attractive, you need to do the things that attract him. So what about your guy? What does he find attractive? What is *the thing* he likes? For one guy I know, it's pink lipstick. Dude just loves pink lipstick. All his wife has to do is to slap some on and his attraction instantly increases. Another guy loves librarian glasses. Just turns him on. Chances are you already know what your husband finds attractive so your next step is to start doing it. Start with a couple of times each week. Fairly simple, yet amazingly effective.

*I know*. During his low T years, you *tried* doing all these things and nothing ever worked. So you just gave up and it kind of ticks you off for me to even suggest that you need to try to attract him again. But here's the deal. The low T years are over. He had a medical issue that he addressed. Could he have addressed it sooner? Sure. But that's water under the bridge.

If you're going to stay in this marriage, you need to do the things that allow it not only to survive, but to *thrive.* You've fixed the general hormone system, now it's time to work on the dopamine system, the one that builds attraction. Now that your husband has the hormones that make it possible for him to experience desire, it's time to do the things that attract him. Every time you do, you increase the positive momentum in the relationship.

## *Let Him Know What Attracts You*

Just as your husband has specific attraction triggers, you also have your own. You need to let him know what they are but there's a bit of

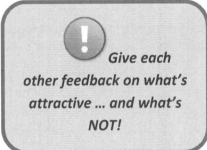

*Give each other feedback on what's attractive … and what's NOT!*

an art to it. You want to do this in a way that doesn't make him feel criticized. The way you approach it is to provide a ton of positive reinforcement when he does that thing that attracts you.

You want to avoid coming across like a drill sergeant telling him what to do. "You never do that <sexy thing> you know I like. You used to do it all the time, but now you never do. You know I like the <sexy thing> but you just don't care enough to attract me." No. Just no. That's not going to work.

Instead, when he does something attractive, you give him positive affirmation. For example, let's say you are really attracted to guys who wear button-down shirts with the sleeves rolled up. There's just something about it that turns you on. The next time he wears a button-down, you're going to tell him how sexy that is. "Wow, you look so hot in that button-down. There's just something about the way you have the sleeves rolled up that turns me on." Be flirty, be sexy. That's what girl game is all about.

### Two-Faced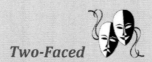

Here's a fun way to let your husband know what attracts you ... and what doesn't. Print a pic of his favorite actress; let's say it's Selma Hayek. Cut it out and mount it on a Popsicle stick. On the other side, tape a picture of someone he finds unattractive; let's say Charlize Theron's character from *Monster*. When your husband does something attractive, flash Selma at him. When he does something unattractive, he gets the homely pic. It's just a light-hearted way to give feedback, and yet it's surprisingly effective.

But beware! It can be a double-edged sword. My husband got into the spirit of it, and now when I do something unattractive, *he* flashes the homely pic at *me*!

## Increase Your Marriage Momentum

In his book, *The Mindful Attraction Plan*, Athol Kay introduces the really useful concept of relationship momentum. The idea is that at any point in time, the energy in your marriage is either increasing or decreasing. Where you start is not as important as whether your momentum is moving upward or downward. No matter where you start, the goal is to do the things that move your marriage in a generally upward direction. This concept is especially helpful in a long-term low T marriage because the energy tends to be very low to begin with.

> **!** *You and your husband are seeing the same interactions through different filters.*

The momentum in your marriage depends on a series of small, daily interactions that you and your spouse perceive as either negative or positive; -1's and +1's. Each interaction in your marriage moves your direction either up or down. Fairly simple concept, right? Keep the positive interactions coming and avoid the negative interactions; the momentum in your marriage improves and the relationship thrives.

The fly in the ointment is that you may not have a clue when your partner is experiencing a -1. We each filter all of our interactions through a lens made up of our past hurts and disappointments, previous interactions with other partners, our own areas of insecurity, individual love language, etc.

It's likely then, that your husband is going to have a wildly disparate view of any given interaction than you do. However, instead of letting you know when he's feeling negative about an interaction, he may hold it all in, assuming that you're purposefully trying to be negative. And resentment builds.

Here's an example from a couple I worked with. The wife had this thing where she would reach over and tweak her husband's nose. Sounds silly I know, but while she meant it to be fun and playful, it drove him nuts. Each time she did it, it was a -1, and with every incident she actually became less attractive to her husband. But because it was such a small thing, he didn't think it was worth mentioning.

Another example, this one from my own marriage. My husband works long hours. Years ago, in an effort to give him time to decompress when he first came home from work, I stopped greeting him at the door. When he walked in, I would look up and smile and ask how his day was, but I would continue doing whatever it was I was doing at the time. I didn't realize it, but it made him feel ... unimportant. As if it didn't matter to me one way or another that he came home from work. Obviously, this wasn't what I intended at all. But the effect was the same. It was just one of those little negative interactions that was diminishing overall satisfaction in the marriage. Not a huge deal, but added up over time it was decreasing our momentum. However, my husband never mentioned any of this to me. Not, that is, until we started tracking our interactions.

## Track Your Interactions

As the two of you work on increasing the momentum in your marriage, you're going to need feedback from each other. Chances are that both of you are missing some of the interactions that affect the energy in your marriage. One helpful tool is to actually track your -1's and +1's.

You'll remember that in Chapter 16 I talked about tracking your marital satisfaction. Tracking your interactions is related, but with a different focus. Tracking your marital satisfaction gives you an overall feel for what's going on in the marriage, while tracking your individual interactions lets you understand the impact your interactions have on that overall marital satisfaction. Kind of a macro view vs. a micro view.

Here's how it works; as you interact with your partner and experience something they say or do as negative, instead of remaining silent about it, you let them know, "Hey, that was a -1."

You may get the same reaction my husband got from me, "Wait. *What*? Not coming to the door to greet you is a -1? *Why*?" As you start to realize that they don't perceive the situation the way you do, the light bulb comes on. "Oh, they aren't trying to be a jerk. We're just seeing this interaction differently."

It's amazing how that defuses the situation and the resentment you're feeling dissipates. It doesn't actually matter whether they understand why you perceive the interaction as negative, although if you use this tool long enough, patterns will gradually emerge that give you a better feel for what triggers your partner. All that matters is that they understand that this was a -1.

During particularly turbulent times in your marriage, it can help to actually keep a chart of your -1's and + 1's and go over them with each other each day. I have honestly been amazed at some of the things my husband has perceived as negative or positive. Things that I never gave a second thought.

A side benefit of this exercise is that you will start understanding your husband's intentions more clearly. You'll both eventually be able to set aside the filters that are creating the negative perceptions to see that your partner isn't trying to hurt you; you simply see things differently. This understanding will allow both of you to start assuming positive intentions instead of immediately jumping to the most negative interpretation of any interaction, something that happens all too frequently in a low T marriage where both attraction and attachment have been affected.

Start tracking your interactions for the next few weeks and see how changing those interactions impacts marital satisfaction for each of you. You should find your momentum improving as you do this. Table 15 gives you some examples of interactions from couples I've worked with.

| Interaction Chart – Husband's Perspective ||
|---|---|
| **+1's** | **-1's** |
| Being fun on date night; looking hot | Playing on your tablet instead of coming to bed |
| Not pulling your hand away from mine when I held it | Acting like I didn't know how to fix the stove |
| Responding playfully to my texts | Criticizing how much time I spend on my job |

Table 15

# Celebrate Your Successes Together

I want you to visualize a team that has just won the play-offs. Picture the excitement and the sense of camaraderie the players share as they lift each other up, give each other high fives, and pour champagne over each other's head. The positive energy simply *pours* out of them ... and it's contagious. Everyone wants to share in the excitement of a winning team.

This is the direction you want your marriage to move toward. Start celebrating each minor success together. This can be simple stuff like achieving a workout goal, or finishing a project on the house. Or bigger things like one of you landing that tough deal, getting a promotion, or reaching a certain financial goal. Or even relational stuff like getting your sex life back on track or going a few weeks without a Death Spiral. Celebrating achievements increases positive energy and builds a sense of being part of a bigger mission.

You can celebrate in all sorts of ways, of course. The classics are going out for dinner, taking a trip together, or having a party. Those are all good things. But you can also build in small celebrations along the way as well.

## *Reward Each Other*

As you and your husband reach the goals you set in your weekly planning meetings, build in some rewards and celebrations. Whether it's going out for a celebration dinner or setting up a new activity you both want to do, take the time to look back and recognize how much you've accomplished and how far you've come. You've worked really hard. Reward yourselves for that.

For one couple I worked with, the wife had a significant weight loss goal. When she hit certain weight milestones, they shopped together for a new outfit for her. For another couple, it was financial debt they were paying down. When they made the last payment, they had a celebration bash. These are the things that increase energy and improve your attachment bonds. They give you a sense of being part of a winning team.

## Accomplishment Board

This is a simple tool, but quite effective. Find an area in your house where you can post each family member's accomplishments. This could be a wall in the kitchen or other shared area. The kids might hang their Honor Roll certificates or a project of which they're especially proud. You and your husband can post goals you've reached with work or things you've accomplished around the house. Take some time each week to celebrate those accomplishments. You could do this at your family meeting, or at dinner each night. Compliment, reward and celebrate. You'll feel the positive energy increase.

# What to Expect at this Point

- *His testosterone levels have probably stabilized by this point, with much fewer ups and downs.*
- *You'll start recognizing how dysfunctional your dynamics became during the low T years.*
- *You'll start creating a 'new normal' as you and your husband change your dynamics.*
- *As your husband takes a stronger role in the family, you'll find yourself second-guessing the way he handles things. This is normal.*
- *It will be hard to trust that this new guy is here to stay. You will find yourself testing him to see if he's strong enough to stand up to you.*
- *Progress will be uneven. There will peaks and valleys in your upward progression. Your heart will sink when he falls back into his old ways. This is all normal. Give it time to solidify.*
- *You will see the momentum in your marriage increase.*
- *You'll find that your attraction for your husband grows and you'll feel more connected to him.*

- *You'll start feeling proud to be married to him.*

# Action Steps

There's a lot to digest in this chapter and a lot of tools that increase attraction. This section has the most action steps, so don't take it all on at once. Just do bite-sized pieces and let your positive momentum grow. When the two of you find your energy flagging, slow the pace down. You've got the rest of your lives together; you'll get there.

- *Set goals together.*
- *Set up a time to go over the family stuff you manage and bring him up to speed.*
- *Meet with each child regularly so your husband knows what's going on in their lives.*
- *Set up weekly planning meetings and start setting goals together.*
- *Play together.*
- *Schedule regular Dopamine Date nights.*
- *Incorporate little dopamine moments into your daily routine.*
- *Work out together.*
- *Remember to be lovers.*
- *Re-connect when you first get home*
- *Take time together before bedtime.*
- *Do the things that attract each other.*
- *Give him positive affirmation when he does something attractive.*
- *Track your interactions.*
- *Celebrate your successes together.*
- *Reward each other.*

# Chapter 19
# Girl Talk
## *Getting the Bedroom Back on Track*

Sex. Ah, therein lies the rub. All through the *Recovery Stage* you've seen progress in many different areas in your marriage, but your sex life continues to lag behind. Sex … or the lack thereof … is the single greatest source of conflict in a low T marriage, and it also takes the longest to get right.

While I've touched on some of the sexual stuff in previous chapters, in this chapter I'm going to go into much more detail because getting the sex right is so important to the healing process. You'll see some overlap in this chapter and the other recovery steps, particularly *Step One,* but this chapter puts it all in one place for you for easy reference. This chapter is designed to help you understand the blockages that are hurting your sex life and give you specific steps for getting the sex you want.

You can't talk about sexual issues without being fairly blunt, so this is where we let our hair down and relax. Picture yourself on the beach with a pitcher of margaritas, hanging out with your girlfriends. Go ahead and kick off your flip flops and get comfortable. No need to be shy, you're amongst friends.

## Life is Passing You By

It's been so long since you've had a good sex life that you don't even remember what it's like. You feel angry and cheated and like your best years are passing you by. The worst times are when you're ovulating; you lie there next to your sleeping husband, your body practically vibrating with need, and you can't figure out how he can remain indifferent. The sound of that peaceful breathing drives you out of your mind! As one woman I worked with said, "He's low T, and I'm nuts!"

You'd never cheat on your husband, but honestly, the temptation is there. Sometimes it takes all you have to walk away instead of flirting with that cute guy at work. You're starved for male attention and admiration, and your husband seems oblivious. Other guys think you're attractive, why doesn't your husband want to toss you on the bed and have his way with you?

## Will It Ever Get Better?

While your husband is feeling better and has more energy and enthusiasm, sex is still … *lackluster*, to put it mildly. You're starting to worry that this is as good as it's going to get.

As I mentioned in Chapter 15, it's normal for the sex life to take a while to get back on track. As your husband gradually adjusts to the higher testosterone levels, you'll probably find that he *talks* about sex a lot more than he actually initiates. There are several reasons for this; changed dynamics in your marriage, lack of confidence, fear of ED, underdeveloped neural pathways, and erratic testosterone levels.

For now, understand that you've just started your recovery process and what is going on now is not indicative of where you'll end up. The burning question in your mind is, "Will it ever get better?"

Yes, it will. It will get better. It's a rollercoaster at first, but it does get better. In fact, it can get amazingly good, better than when you first met, but it's going to take some effort and some patience.

## He's the Hunter, You're the Prey

In Chapter 16, I discussed that your husband was most likely neutral about sex when his T levels initially went down. While he didn't have high desire, he wasn't actually negative about sex; it simply never crossed his mind. Over time, though, all of that changed. The less he initiated, the more

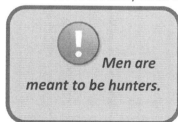

*Men are meant to be hunters.*

you took over. This was completely normal; however, the more you pushed for sex, the more defensive and prickly he became. This substantially changed the dynamics in your marriage in ways you didn't understand or intend.

Men are meant to be hunters. The thrill of the chase gives them the dopamine they need to stay sexually alert. Without the chase, they tend to lose interest. Now obviously, when his T levels were low, he wasn't going to chase so you had to. Now that his general hormones are back where they should be, it's time to turn all this around. I'll give you some tools to do this later in the chapter.

## Lack of Confidence

Another piece of the puzzle is that guys who have had low T usually struggle with confidence, not surprising given that testosterone fuels confidence and boldness. This lack of confidence lingers even after the T levels have been addressed. The only 'cure' is time and practice. He simply needs time to redevelop his sexual confidence. The more supportive you are during this time period, the better.

I know you've been sex-deprived for a long time. I know that you want that bold, confident lover back. You're ready for him to go all caveman on you and throw you on the bed and have his way with you. That will all come, but not quite yet.

## Fear of ED/PE

This is an issue that can't be over-stated. When a guy has struggled with ED (erectile dysfunction) or PE (premature ejaculation), it

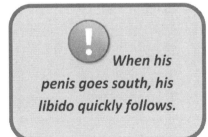

*When his penis goes south, his libido quickly follows.*

completely shoots his confidence. It takes him a long time to regain it, even once his equipment is working again.

If your guy is still struggling with ED, he will feel emasculated and be quite reluctant to initiate and experience the possible humiliation of a penis that doesn't work. He's going to have to address that before the two of you can make progress in the bedroom.

Even if your husband's erections are reliable again now that he's on T therapy, understand that some remnants of the old fear will remain. He may also have developed some habits that allowed him to work around the lack of erections before, but that are unnecessary and even detrimental now.

> ***PIV = Penis in Vagina:  Another term for intercourse***
>
> ***PE = Premature Ejaculation:  He finishes too soon.***

## Coping Mechanisms for ED

For example, a guy with ED often skips over foreplay and gets right down to it. The reason for this, of course, is that he's afraid his penis will stop working. There's no time for him to stop and enjoy your body or notice your sexy lingerie because he's afraid he'll lose his erection. He may also skip the lube for fear that his erection won't last long enough to apply it. Everything centers on the performance anxiety he's feeling.

If this is the case for your husband, he may ask for blowjobs or hand jobs instead of PIV because the firmer pressure makes it easier for him to keep his erection. This is disappointing for you when what you're really wanting from him is a hard pounding!

One woman's husband figured out that if she tightened her legs around him and held perfectly still, he could hold his erection. The only problem with this was that she couldn't feel anything in this position except friction, and had started to dread the rug burn she was getting. Obviously, not ideal circumstances for satisfying sex.

A typical coping mechanism for a guy who's concerned about erections is that he'll initiate exclusively in the morning. That's when his T levels are higher and his erections are more reliable. The trouble with this is that mornings are usually not conducive to good sex. You're rushed with the need to get the kids to school and then get to work on time. Sex in the morning is often less than satisfying for you, but that's the only time he initiates.

> *"My wife mentioned that it's been a long time since we've had sex, but I just have no interest in embarrassing myself by starting something I probably can't finish."*
>
> *--Chris, 39, Finance Mgr.*

Another common response is denial. When a guy is struggling with ED, he will frequently ignore it or pretend it's not happening. He may blame it on you, telling you that you're 'just not as tight as you used to be'. This may hurt and infuriate you, but it's fairly typical.

I talked to one guy who was going to suggest surgery to his wife to correct her 'lack of tightness' until I suggested to him that he try Viagra to see if it helped *before* he talked to his wife. *Whew!* Critical moment averted.

Here's one woman's account of her husband's reaction to ED:

> *"It drives me crazy when my husband loses his erection but pretends it's not happening. He just ignores it and keeps pumping away as if everything is fine. Why does he do this? We both know it's not working.*
>
> *I guess he's hoping that the stimulation will help his erection come back, but it never does.*
>
> *I wish he would just use his Cialis! He said he doesn't think he really needs it anymore! Argh!"*
>
> *--Jill, 49, Accountant*

## Get It In Before Nine

Related to this is the way he'll be all over you early in the day when sex is off the table because of kids and work. You're lying in bed in the morning and he's rubbing against you, pushing himself into you, telling you how much he needs you. Now obviously, you both know that nothing's going to happen in the moment, so you take a raincheck. Except ... he never cashes in the raincheck. By that night, you're raring to go, having thought about him all day ... but he's all droopy-eyed, slouching around, yawning. *And all the old feelings of rejection come pouring back in.*

You've started thinking this is some mind game he's playing, that maybe he has all these deep issues and resentments that stop him from carrying through with the morning's promises. Nope. It's much simpler than that. Testosterone levels are at their highest in the morning, supplying him with the energy and libido he needs to initiate. They gradually wane over the course of the day to their lowest point late at night. In addition, morning erections are the most reliable. By 11pm when the two of you actually get into bed, he's wiped. Energizer Bunny ran out of gas.

So the trick is to have sex as early in the day as possible. Get those kids to bed early and hightail it to the bedroom. Do not pass Go, do not collect $200. Just straight to the bedroom. Again, this is a temporary measure and will pass as his energy levels pick up.

## Lousy Sex

Both of you have probably picked up multiple coping strategies over the years of ED/low T/PE. He's done lame initiations for a long time because he lacked confidence/was afraid his penis wouldn't work/was too tired. You've been willing to accept any type of sex he's willing to throw your way because you needed sex/wanted to attract him/were desperate for connection. While those coping strategies got you both through some very lean years, they're actively hurting your marriage at this point.

You are still operating from a scarcity mindset, where sex comes few and far between, and you have to take what you can get. You may be so grateful that he is finally beginning to have an interest in sex again that you fall all over yourself to give him what he wants. "Finally," you think, "he wants me. I need to turn him on and not make any demands on him that might turn him off again."

You're afraid that if you set reasonable sexual boundaries with your husband, he'll go back to the dark years where he ignored you sexually. You feel that in order keep him interested, you need to respond to him as soon as he shows interest.

You need to understand though, that if you fall back on the bed, ready and willing anytime he glances your way, he will lose attraction for you. Let me say it again … if you are higher drive than he is, and he can have you on a whim, he will want you less. That's a lot to take in, I know. But as I mentioned in Chapter 16, by nature the male of the species typically chases the female. When that dynamic changes in a low T marriage, it hurts attraction.

Think back to when you first met. Chances are he's the one who pursued you. He saw you as a prize to be won and that piqued his interest in you. He chased, you ran, and you eventually let him catch you. All was good. Now ask yourself; if back then you had accepted any type of sexual overture he had offered, no matter how lame, would he have continued to pursue you? Or would your failure to demonstrate value have lowered his attraction for you?

Make sure to set reasonable boundaries around sex. If you want lube, make sure he uses it. If you need more foreplay, let him know. If a certain position works for him but doesn't work for you, then change it up. It will be awkward at first, but it's necessary to change all these negative dynamics.

It took Cindy a while to learn to set reasonable expectations:

*"For the last couple of weeks, Allen's been working too hard to have the energy to initiate. I'm trying to keep things on track, so last week I gave him a blowjob. He loved it, but no orgasm for me.*

*I initiated two times this week and he turned me down. The third time, he was interested and we started having really great sex. I couldn't believe how hot it was and how into it he was.*

*He was saying all these sexy things in my ear, and I was getting so excited … but then he finished before I could orgasm! I couldn't believe it! It's been three weeks for me and he knows I'm to the point of going out of my mind. Why would he do that? And of course, as soon as he finished, he fell asleep, which is what he always does. I lay awake for hours, and now I feel so angry with him, I could kill him!*

*Every time I think we're getting on track sexually, something seems to happen to throw us off."*

## Stop Having Quickies

I've worked with some women who just kept giving their husband orgasm after orgasm through blowjobs or hand jobs without getting anything in return. When a woman does this, she is engaging in a covert contract that if she pleases him, then he will want to please her; however, he's not privy to the covert contract, so it all blows up in her face. Then she is angry and resentful toward him for days afterwards. It's a dysfunctional and damaging dynamic, but it's common in recovering low T marriages. If you're doing this with your husband, you are showing low value. You are training him that he doesn't need to expend any effort in order to attract you. Is this the message you want to convey to him?

You need to stop giving him gratuitous blowjobs/hand jobs/quickies while getting nothing for yourself. If it's been five days since you've had an orgasm, and he asks you for a blowjob and you comply, knowing that it will be another five days before he shows an interest again, you are not doing the marriage any favors. You are simply training him to do lousy initiations, and you are actually lowering his attraction for you.

> ***Covert contract - when someone does something for someone else without explaining what they want in return.***

One woman I worked with had a tough time with this. Every request from her husband was met with immediate acquiescence. If he wanted a blowjob or a hand job, she was there. But then she would resent the fact that he wasn't reciprocating. She had a covert contract where she assumed that if she met his sexual needs, he would meet hers. The problem was that he wasn't privy to her assumption. All he saw was a wife who did whatever he wanted. She had trained him to disregard her sexual needs. Over time, she actually became less attracted to him because of the resentment.

She felt that if she rejected his sexual requests, he would stop being attracted to her but, in reality, the opposite was actually true. By not setting standards, she was diminishing his attraction along with her own. Once she started setting reasonable sexual boundaries, he became much more interested in her, and she regained attraction for him.

You don't need to satisfy your husband's every sexual desire immediately in order to create attraction. You want him to keep that sexual hunger for you. Let him have the thrill of the chase, he'll desire you more.

While this dynamic is important during the whole *Recovery Stage*, it is especially important in *Step One,* when you are actively working to stop the behaviors that are creating negative energy.

## Striking a Balance

There's a bit of a balance you have to strike here. While you don't want to accept lousy sex that's easy for him but unsatisfying for you, you also don't want to be critical of his initiations and performance, causing him to shut down and withdraw.

People learn best in low-stress environments. Remember how stress shuts down neuroplasticity - the brain's ability to reorganize its neural pathways? Keep the bedroom low stress so that your husband feels comfortable initiating with you. Encourage him with words and actions when he does the things that attract and arouse you. You don't need to be a drill sergeant, but lightly encouraging him, "Oh yes, that feels so good," or "Mmmm.... do that again. That felt wonderful," goes a long way toward motivating him to repeat an action. Or even a simple, "Here feels better," as you move his hand.

Remember that we're all training each other all the time. Set healthy boundaries by encouraging the stuff that improves your sex life, and discouraging the stuff that hurts it. Sounds pretty simple when you put it that way, doesn't it?

## Temporarily Losing Attraction

As I mentioned briefly in Chapter 15, it is quite common for a woman in a low T marriage to eventually lose attraction for her husband. A husband with low T has usually stopped displaying the masculine traits that attract a woman. In addition, the attachment bond between them has diminished considerably because of the lack of sex and the repeated sexual rejection the wife has experienced. All of this takes its toll on attraction.

It usually works like this; when a woman's husband first loses interest in sex, it motivates her to try harder to attract him. She starts working out, dresses nicer, tries new lingerie, incorporates new sexy moves, etc. She's convinced that the problem is her and so she knocks herself out trying to get his interest.

Over time, though, the other shoe drops and she realizes that nothing she tries is going to work. At this point, she normally gets furious, completely loses attraction for him and stops wanting sex. She tends to freak out a bit when this happens because she's afraid that her sex drive is broken, but this is a normal part of the low T script.

In a strange way, it can actually be helpful when she loses her desire for her husband. All of these years, she has put pressure on him to be more sexual with her, and he's become highly resistant to this sexual pressure.

What happens is that when her attraction wanes, she stops putting pressure on him for sex and may actually turn him down once in a while. While this initially takes him aback, it also takes the sexual pressure off him and frees him to become more of the aggressor.

As long as it's not carried too far, this change in dynamics increases his attraction in the long term.

## He Feels Entitled

The first few times that he initiates and you're not interested, it's going to rock his world … and not in a good way. Because he's been lower desire than you all this time, it's been *years* since he's had to expend any effort in order to attract you. In fact, it's possible that he's actively tried to dissuade you from wanting sex with him.

You've trained him for years that he only has to look your way and you'll be there ready to go. He is so used to you being the pursuer that he simply can't comprehend that you're turning him down and he may react quite badly. In fact, it's very possible that he will stop initiating for a while. That's okay, it's a necessary restructuring of the whole sexual dynamic between the two of you.

Simply let him know that while you *want* to want sex, you're having a hard time getting there and you need his help. Over time, he'll gain confidence and his initiations will grow stronger. As he starts doing the things that attract you, you will find your desire returning.

## Refractory Period

One woman learned about her husband's refractory period the hard way. She and her husband had a special weekend lined up at a swanky

resort. They had a date planned at a luau and were dressed to kill. She had visions of tropical drinks with little pink umbrellas and then coming home to a long, leisurely lovemaking session. Unfortunately, they started the evening by having a quickie on the sofa before they left, and that was it for the night. While she was just revving up, he was finished.

What she didn't take into account is that most guys have a **refractory period**, or recovery phase, after sex where they become much less interested in, and even less able to have sex again. What happens is that when you and your husband have sex, dopamine and oxytocin levels gradually rise, eventually peaking at the point of orgasm. After orgasm, both dopamine and oxytocin drop sharply. In addition, testosterone receptors also decrease and prolactin levels rise, leading to a dramatic drop in sexual interest. This is a feature, not a bug.

The drop is much more pronounced in guys with low T, and their refractory periods tend to last much longer, sometimes as long as two or three weeks. As his T levels stabilize and he becomes more sexual, this refractory period usually shortens. When my husband was in the dark years of low T, it typically took him weeks to be interested in sex again. Over time, his refractory period has shortened to just a day or two at the most. Sometimes he's ready before I am! If you had told me that a few years ago, I would have laughed in disbelief.

This explains why your husband can stalk you like a lion stalks a gazelle, and then immediately after sex, you become invisible to him. That's actually normal. It's not some deep-rooted emotional issue; it's simply hormones. It's just that it lasts longer in low T guys.

If, as soon as your husband expresses the slightest bit of interest, you satisfy his sexual desire with a quick orgasm, you will never get the intense desire from him you are looking for.

# Ovulation

It's also worth noting that women normally have a sharp spike in desire around the time they ovulate. This is the time when a woman craves a higher level of intensity, desire and leadership from her husband and often feels angry when she doesn't get it.

During the early days of the *Recovery Stage* when your husband is still not fully sexual, you're going to want to plan some exciting activities that don't involve him during ovulation. Otherwise, it's easy to go out of your mind wanting something he can't yet give you.

## Desiring Desire

What you're starting to realize is that even though his libido has increased and he seems to want sex more frequently, there's still something missing. His erections have gotten better and he seems to enjoy sex while it's happening, but ……..

Where's that raw, heart-pounding passion that he used to have? Where is the *'I've just got to have you'* guy he used to be? Why does he wait for you to initiate instead of jumping you when you get home? You also wonder why you aren't happier now that you're getting more sex. After all, that's what you've said you've been wanting all these years.

There's a little secret about being a wife in a low T marriage. The secret is that it's not about sex; it's all about desire. Yeah, I know. That takes a few minutes to absorb, doesn't it?

It's not really about sex. If it were, you'd be fine with your *Mr. Friendly* vibrator and a few double A's. The wife in a low T marriage could possibly live without sex. Sex plays into it, of course. There are those nights where you lie next to him, aching and throbbing and all you really want is a hard pounding. But that's just a small portion of it. After all, there are multiple ways to get an orgasm.

What you're needing, what you're craving, what you can't live without is ….. *desire*. It undergirds every single action on your part. Every time you blow up at your husband because he didn't initiate in just the right way, or he wasn't dominant enough, or he initiated but he didn't seem into it … every single time, what you needed from him was desire.

Sometimes you feel like there's not enough desire in the world to fill you up. That if he spent every waking moment for the next 37 years showing his desire for you, it still wouldn't be enough. But that's not true. Once he actually learns to consistently show his desire for you, you will be surprised at how quickly that void in you is filled.

It's tricky at first because he's so inconsistent. He shows desire for three days, you finally have sex, he goes through his refractory period, and then nothing for the next four days. Or he feels criticized by you, the two of you go into a Death Spiral and he turns into a eunuch for the next seven days. Every time this happens, you feel like you're starting over. So there's a work-around that helps you get past all that. *Edging*.

# Edging

*Edging* refers to the practice of someone, usually the guy, deliberately engaging in sexual stimulation without finishing to orgasm. Here's why it's important in a low T marriage; when your husband is sexually stimulated, even if it doesn't lead to an orgasm, it increases his testosterone levels. It also strengthens the sexual pathways in his brain that he's trying to develop. The more he

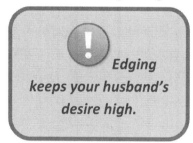

*Edging keeps your husband's desire high.*

thinks about sex, touches you, gets erections, etc., the quicker those pathways can develop. The touching leads to oxytocin, and the sexual excitement increases dopamine.

Edging increases both attraction and attachment. Two birds with one stone. The more often you get sexual with each other, the better off you are. In other words, you need to fool around more. He needs to frequently get all hot and heavy without finishing. Kind of like high school all over again.

You, on the other hand, can have as many orgasms as you want … or are capable of. Now isn't that the nicest thing you've heard all day?

# A Day of Edging

So, what would a day of edging look like? You'd start in the morning when his testosterone levels are high and his erections are naturally strongest. In the past, maybe you would ignore his attempts at *nudge nudge, poke poke* because you knew there wasn't time for much to happen. The kids are due to come running in, the alarm's going to ring, and there's no way you're going to get off. And there's no way you want him to finish by himself again because you know it will be another long week before he shows any interest.

With edging, all of that is different. You fool around a little and feel more connected. His sexual interest is piqued. You can have an orgasm if there's time and you want to, but he doesn't finish. Oxytocin and dopamine are both on the rise. Your connection and attraction grow.

Later that day, when you get home from work, you take some time to reconnect in your bedroom. You kiss, you hug, and maybe you tease him a bit. Maybe he gets an erection, maybe not. But his interest and his dopamine increase. By bedtime, his desire is growing and you have sex together. You finish, but he holds off. Rinse and repeat for a day or two until he decides to have an orgasm and starts the cycle over again.

Edging is really helpful for a low T couple. It's a temporary workaround as you repair your marriage, and at some point it goes by the wayside. For now though, it's an excellent tool to add to your recovery arsenal. It keeps his desire revved up and his interest in you keen. Which brings me to another point ...

## In You or On You

The whole point of edging is to keep his sexual interest *in you* at a peak. That's not going to happen if he's having sex by himself. It's quite common for a low T guy to use porn and/or masturbation rather than having sex with his partner. At first, that seems surprising ... if his libido is low, why would he want to masturbate to porn? ... but when you think about it, it's actually very logical.

Most low T guys struggle with energy and confidence. A lot of them are dealing with ED or PE. Masturbation/porn is the seemingly perfect solution to his problem. The mental stimulation from porn delivers huge amounts of dopamine with very little effort and it takes a lot less energy to have virtual sex than it does to have real life sex. In addition, with masturbation he can relax and not worry about his wife rejecting his initiation or about whether he's good enough to satisfy her in bed.

There's also the physical stimulation factor. Because his hand can create a tighter grip than a woman's vagina, ED is not as much of a problem, and because he doesn't have to worry about lasting long enough to bring his wife to orgasm, any problems with PE disappear as well.

*"When we do have sex, it's okay, but nowhere near as intense as it used to be. I still occasionally masturbate to porn, but sex with my wife just feels like too much work."*
**--Dave, 36, Software Designer**

The fly in the ointment, of course, is that his masturbation/porn use keeps the two of you from having sex together. The stark reality is that he has a limited amount of sexual energy, especially in the early stages of T therapy. If he's expending it anywhere other than you, it's a problem. He simply has to knock it off.

Don't blow up at him. Let him know that you understand that he's tempted, but at the same time, let him know that directing his sexual energy outside of the marriage is not okay. This is where you need to set a reasonable boundary with him ... if he has sex, it needs to be in you or on you. Anything else is a deal breaker.

## The Most Important Ingredient

The most important factor in getting your sex life back on track is *patience*. This is not a quick process for most low T couples and the longer he's been dealing with low T, the longer the recovery process. Things didn't get bad overnight, and they're not going to get better overnight either.

You need to pace yourself. It's going to take time for both of you to change your brain patterns and overcome all the dysfunctional dynamics you've developed over the years. Be gentle with yourself and with him. You've got years and years to enjoy a great sex life together. You'll get there!

# What to Expect at this Point

- *Sometimes you'll feel like a cat on a hot tin roof as you wait for his sex drive to catch up to his hormones.*

- *There will be times where it will seem like you're making no progress at all.*
- *There will be times where you will feel hopeless and it will take all you have to avoid a Death Spiral.*
- *You will most likely find yourself falling back into old patterns where you pursue him. That's okay, it's tough to change your brain.*
- *His initiations will likely be fairly lame for a while. You may get a lot of morning nudge nudge, poke poke initiations. This will change as his confidence grows. He will not always follow up on those morning initiations because he is still struggling with energy and libido in the evenings.*
- *You will probably struggle not to accept lousy sex because you are so used to having to take whatever he offers. This will improve as you practice setting boundaries.*
- *His refractory period will most likely be fairly long at first, but should shorten over time.*
- *You may find yourself wanting more even after a session of great sex. It's likely that what you're really wanting is not more sex, you're actually wanting more desire from him. Edging will help in that area.*
- *If he's used porn in the past, he may fall back on that as an easy fix.*
- *There will probably be times where you don't feel all that attracted to him. That's normal. As he changes his behaviors, your attraction will return.*
- *He will most likely not be at all happy when you fail to respond to a lame initiation. He's been a bit spoiled all these years. Over time his initiations will improve. It is likely be a bit of a rollercoaster as the two of you adjust this dynamic and reach a new equilibrium.*

# Action Steps

- *Stay hopeful; understand that you're rebuilding from the ground up and you're going to have growing pains.*
- *Stop pursuing him and give him the chance to be The Hunter.*
- *Understand that his lack of confidence will cause him to act in less than productive ways. Don't take it personally because most of it comes from his own insecurities and has nothing to do with you.*
- *Recognize that if he's struggled with ED or PE in the past, it has taken a tremendous hit on his confidence levels. It will take him a while to get past this.*
- *Try to have sex as early at night as possible, or even in the daytime if you get the chance. These are the times when his testosterone levels, confidence and sexual performance are all at their peak.*
- *Set reasonable sexual standards. No more sex that's easy for him but lousy for you.*
- *Strike a good balance. While you don't want to accept lousy sex, you also don't want to be critical and discourage him from even trying.*
- *Set a firm boundary about him directing his sexual energy into any source other than you. In you or on you is the order of the day.*
- *Expect some turbulence as his sex drive increases and you find your balance. It will eventually settle into the new normal.*

# Chapter 20
# Just When You Thought It Was Safe ...
### *The Set-Back*

... to go back in the water.

Congratulations! You made it to the end of *Stage Four*. *Woo Hoo*! You and your husband are getting along well, his T levels are finally nice and stable, the two of you are working and playing together, having a lot of fun, and the sex is great and steadily gaining momentum. *Ahhh*. Life is good.

But then .... he does it. The thing. He does the thing again. He stops taking his meds, forgets to order the Cialis, stops initiating, hits the porn again, whatever. There are numerous variations but it's that thing that drives you crazy and that you simply can't live with.

Suddenly, everything comes to a screeching halt and you feel like you've been hit by a truck. This is the point where you're going to feel completely defeated and you're going to want to give up. Don't.

In this chapter, I cover the inevitable back tracking that's part of the low T script and how you can navigate it as quickly and easily as possible without losing too much forward momentum.

The inevitable setback is an integral part of the Low T script. I see it over and over again with the guys I work with. He'll be making steady progress, doing well with the T therapy, feeling great about his improved erections, initiating steadily and building attraction with his wife, but then at some point he falters and everything blows up.

It used to take me by surprise, but I've come to expect it. The conversation tends to follow the same track each time:

## Conversation from the Low T Script

*"So, how are things going?"*

*"Uh, not so well."*

*"Mmm hmmm. So what happened? You stop taking your T therapy/Viagra/Cialis?"*

*"Yeah! How'd you know?"*

*"Lucky guess."*

# Magical Thinking

I used to be stumped as to what was going on with this, but I've come to realize that everyone engages in magical thinking. It's extremely difficult for an individual to accept that they need a medicine in order to feel good.

I experienced the same dynamic when my thyroid started acting up. I put off taking thyroid meds for six months because I was determined not to be a 'person who takes meds'. It seemed like an admission of weakness to me. You see this same phenomenon in people who are taking psyche meds, even when the meds make the difference in having a normal life or a life of chaos. It's normal to feel this way.

# Door #1 is Forever Closed

What helped me get past the denial and to a point of acceptance was realizing that I wanted something that was no longer available. Behind Door #1 was the pipe dream where my thyroid was functioning as it should and I felt as good as I did when I was 20 without any type of medical intervention. I kept pretending that Door #1 was still open, but it wasn't.

Door #2 was the real world where my thyroid had gone wonky and I was tired and unmotivated, felt cold all the time, and was having a hard time maintaining my normal weight. I insisted on picking Door #2 while pretending that it was Door #1.

I had to admit to myself that Door #1 was closed before I could finally move on to Door #3. Behind Door #3 was a life where I took my thyroid meds and had all those 'horrible' side effects of increased energy, thick shiny hair, improved libido and a metabolism that burned calories efficiently. I had to accept that my body was no longer operating the way I wanted it to, but that I was pretty darned lucky to be able to supplement my depleted thyroid hormone with a cheap, easy-to-take pill.

Your guy also has to reach a level of acceptance in order to truly move on. As do you. I've seen plenty of women who hate the idea that their husband has 'something wrong with him' and they hang on to the fantasy that the low T is magically going to disappear.

Both of you have to give up the magical thinking. Door #1 is closed and you have two choices left; either Door #2 where your husband has all the low T symptoms that make him feel like crap, or Door #3 where he can take a readily-available med and feel pretty wonderful. It's a clear choice.

## Conversations from Out in the Field

This is how it played out for Laura:

*"He has been dragging his feet on the testosterone. He said that he's just waiting on the pharmacy, but we've had that script for three months! When we first got the prescription, I told him I'd be glad to order it for him but he said he wanted to handle it himself. Sex has dropped to once every two weeks. Great, right back where we started."*

*-- Laura, 53, Radiologist*

And for Jennifer:

*"He's stopped initiating again. For once, I didn't fall apart. I stayed calm and simply asked him, 'Okay, what's up? You can beat around the bush or just come out with the truth.'*

*He admitted that his Cialis script ran out three weeks ago, so he decided to see if he still needed it. He didn't want to go through the hassle of making a doctor appointment to get the Cialis renewed. And, of course, he's not having erections anymore.*

*After all the work I've put into fixing this problem and he can't take the time to make a lousy doctor appointment? I am so pissed!*

*We haven't had sex for three weeks! I can't go back to living this way. I can't stay with him if this is as good as it's going to get."*

*– Jennifer, 40, Programmer*

And how it looks from the guy's standpoint:

*"I did feel better on the testosterone but then I wondered if it was all in my head. You know, like a placebo effect. So I stopped taking it just to see if it really made a difference.*

*I felt okay for a week or two, but then my energy tanked, and before I knew it, two weeks went by with no sex. My wife is devastated because she thinks I am purposely sabotaging our marriage. I'm not; I just hate being dependent on some drug to make me a man."*

# Hope for the Best, Plan for the Worst

When the inevitable happens and he makes a misstep, knowing about it ahead of time is going to make a huge difference. It turns it into a little blip instead of a nuclear explosion.

There are a few do's and don'ts when he stops initiating. You're going to be tempted to try and 'have it out with him'. You'll want to ask him why he's not initiating, whether he's mad at you, whether he's not attracted, etc. Don't.

> **!** *He's going to stop taking his meds at some point. It's part of the Low T script.*

You probably won't get any clear answers because he will feel put on the spot. He'll likely go into defensive mode where he throws out plausible reasons that may or may not have anything to do with the truth. He really doesn't want to admit to you that he's stopped taking his meds, so instead he's going to throw out a huge smokescreen.

Instead, what you need to do is approach this quite calmly and directly. You need to ask him simple questions without being accusatory.

*Your first step* is to ask him if he's out of Viagra/Cialis/Levitra. You would be amazed at the number of guys who stop initiating for no reason other than that they forgot to order the Cialis or it took longer than expected to be delivered, etc. They end up not initiating simply because they're afraid the equipment isn't going to work.

*After that*, if he responds that he has a supply of Cialis, et al., the next step is to ask him if he's actually taking it. It does him no good if it sits in the bottle. You may get a shame-faced response that he wanted to see if he could do without it.

*Next*, if you eliminate the first two possibilities, check to see if he's been sticking to his T therapy. Most guys will stop using testosterone at some point just to see if their body will kick back in and produce it.

When things are going smoothly, they tend to get a false sense of complacency and stop taking their T.

**The next thing** is to ask him to draw some labs and see where his T levels are. He may be converting too much testosterone into estrogen, or if he's using a gel or cream, his body may have stopped absorbing it. It's also possible that his internal production has shut down and his total T has decreased.

**Another possibility is that his energy levels have dropped** for some reason. Look at sleep patterns and unusual sources of stress.

**Finally,** the last thing to check is whether he's resorted to porn. This is common when a guy's energy level drops. Porn is easy and a stress-reliever for a lot of guys. If he was a frequent user in the past, his first reaction in times of stress may be to go back to porn.

Once you identify the problem, you have to have a clear idea of how you're going to respond. Think about your response ahead of time so that you don't make snap decisions. While you don't want to blow up, you do need to set clear boundaries about what you will and will not accept in a marriage.

## Set Reasonable Boundaries

It is a *reasonable* expectation that your husband will treat a diagnosed medical condition that is affecting his health and his marriage. It is also reasonable to expect that he will treat any ED issues he has. One thing that seems to help a guy feel more comfortable with this is to refer to Cialis, et al. as a 'performance enhancer' instead of 'your ED meds'. Guys usually hate to take meds, whereas they generally tend to enjoy enhancing their performance.

It's also more than reasonable to have an 'in me or on me' policy. As I mentioned earlier, it's not okay for him to deprive you of sex because he's off having it by himself. It's fine to set that boundary with him.

You need to recognize your own value in this marriage. After all, you have stuck by him and been loyal when some women wouldn't have been. You have done a boatload of research and work to help him address a medical issue. You are a woman of value. Be sure to act like it.

## False Defeat

While you will probably feel as if all your combined efforts have been for nothing, you need to understand that while this situation is a setback, it's not actually a defeat. It is a normal part of the low T script and if you respond productively, it can actually strengthen both you and the marriage in general.

Your reaction is quite important as a show of high value. You need to be able to respond strongly without blowing up. Knowing what to expect gets you most of the way there.

# What to Expect at this Point

- *Everything will be going along amazingly well, the relationship is good, sex is great, when all of a sudden … BAM … it all falls apart.*
- *He will stop taking his meds at some point. I've never seen it fail.*
- *You are probably going to take it personally, as if he doesn't care about you. That's not the case; he's just engaging in Magical Thinking.*
- *You are going to feel like blowing up. It's okay to be angry, you just have to channel that anger productively.*
- *When you ask him what's going on, he may try to dance around the truth. He feels like an idiot for stopping the meds.*

# Action Steps

- *Stay calm and don't explode.*
- *Ask him direct questions about the meds/porn use/etc. Keep them factual instead of emotional.*

- *Set firm boundaries with him. It's not okay for him to ignore a medical condition. You are not willing to live in a sexless marriage. This is a deal breaker.*
- *State your expectations: he stays on his T therapy, he uses Cialis if he needs it and he follows an 'in you or on you' policy.*
- *Accept this as a temporary blip in an otherwise successful recovery.*

# Stage Five

# High T Marriage

"Are you going to pour yourself another margarita?" my husband asked me.

I looked at him questioningly. I wasn't much of a drinker and he knew it. We were staying in for New Year's Eve, so I had bought the stuff to make margaritas, but I rarely had more than one.

He came up behind me and put his arms around me. "I want you loose for tonight, I have plans," he said quietly into my ear. I could feel him smiling.

Plans? That sounded mildly alarming …. but intriguing. I looked back at him out of the corner of my eye and blushed. I still wasn't used to this bold new man who talked so openly about what he wanted.

I thought back to our previous New Year's Eves and it was hard to believe that this was the same guy who would watch a movie with the kids and fall asleep on the sofa long before midnight. What a difference a year of T therapy had made!

After getting ready for bed, I walked out of the bath and into the bedroom. My husband looked me over approvingly and then pulled me down on top of him on the bed, running his hands over the lace of my outfit.

"Mmmmm ….. I like this," he said. "It covers and reveals all at the same time." His hands started arranging my body on the bed. "Okay, I want you to stay just like this while I brush my teeth."

"This is business, ma'am, strictly business. Just doing my job here," he said as he moved my legs a bit. He stepped back and admired his work. "Stay right there. No moving."

He continued watching me as he brushed, scolding me when I moved or complained. It was obvious how much he was enjoying the game .... and the view.

Where had this bold, confident man come from? I hadn't seen him for years! It was like all the layers of Low T that had covered up the real him for so long were being wiped away in front of my eyes.

I had always been attracted to him, but never like this. Now he knew all the buttons to push, and when he chose to push them, my mind and body reacted without me even thinking about it.

He rejoined me and put his 'plans' into action. Everything flowed seamlessly together, with nothing seeming to take any effort. I felt completely connected to him and everything we did felt ... right.

I had wanted this for so long. The sense of togetherness and connection. Where his actions and my actions came together with no conscious thought. Nothing choreographed, nothing planned. Just a smooth blending of two people.

As we neared midnight, we could hear the fireworks going off outside. Someone was having a huge celebration nearby. I was just grateful for our own personal celebration inside.

# Chapter 21
# Uncharted Territory
### *You Can't Go Back*

Welcome to *Stage Five*! You've had a long journey and overcome a lot of obstacles to get here. Now that you've arrived, let's talk about what you can expect. After all, this is uncharted territory for your marriage; while you've lived life *without* low T, you've never experienced life *after* low T!

 For better or worse, you and your husband are not the same people you were before you started down this path and your marriage is not the same marriage. Practically speaking, you will find that you have more sex, more energy, more strength, more peace, and more time than you had during the low T years.

Emotionally, you will also find that the ways in which you and your husband relate to each other have changed. The journey has changed your marriage and your family, it's changed you and your husband as individuals, and it's also changed the make-up of your daily lives together.

## The Marriage Has Changed

*You argue less.* During the low T years, arguments were frequent but not productive, just round and round the same resentment treadmill. Once a couple resolves the core conflict caused by the hormonal issue, arguments become less frequent and resolve more quickly because the underlying anger is gone. You stop having those Death Spirals that last for weeks.

*You simply have more fun together*. You stop that deadly dynamic where you are parents first and foremost. Instead, you become lovers who are also parenting together. That means that you allow yourselves to go out and do exciting things together. You give your marriage priority. You remember what you liked about each other in the first place.

***You look forward to seeing him.*** Low T drains a man's energy so much that it can be exhausting to be around him. Once his energy levels rebound, you find yourself happy to hear his footsteps and eager to see him again; you once again feel that little thrill of anticipation. Why, *hello* old friend, I've missed you.

> **!** *You and your husband are different people now.*

***Sex becomes more frequent and more exciting***. You'll find yourself trying new things and being more candid with each other about sex. You were forced to communicate about sex during the low T years in ways you never had to before and the resulting openness has become part of your new dynamic. *Good-bye, roommate*; I will miss you not!

***You start working together as a team***, maybe for the first time. You communicate with each other about what's going on with the house, the kids, the careers, and the marriage. The weekly planning meetings have given you the tool and the time to share information, and it pays off well.

***You feel an increased sense of connection.*** Because of the effect Low T has on attachment and bonding, couples often feel little sense of connection to each other and even see each other as 'the enemy'. Once his libido reappears and the sex comes back, feelings of love and empathy rebound for both of you.

***You become much more mindful*** of the need to actively attract each other and more aware of the specifics that increase attraction for your partner. You approach your marriage and sex life much more consciously than you ever did before. Before the low T years, your marriage ran on autopilot to a certain extent. You knew what worked and what didn't work and you were able to be complacent.

Overcoming this struggle together forced you to take your relationship apart and examine it and decide that it was worth fighting for; the low T years actually brought your marriage to a better place in the end.

## Your Husband Has Changed

Low T is a life-changing experience for a man. He doesn't simply go back to being the man he was before he had low T.

*He puts a higher value on his health.* Every man has to face his own mortality sooner or later. With Low T, that moment comes sooner rather than later. In general, men tend to take their health for granted. For many men, they may not even see a doctor all through their 20's and 30's, and even into their 40's. My husband calls it 'young man mindset'. They tend to scoff at getting annual physicals and they count on their bodies to keep running with no maintenance. Low T changes all that.

Once a guy goes through the low T fog and comes out on the other side, he normally becomes much more conscious of living well. He starts eating healthier, gets more sleep, cuts down on excessive alcohol, etc. He'll start working out, maybe picks up a martial art or new sport. He lives his life more intensely. It's like he wants to grab on to his new-found energy and strength and squeeze every drop out of it.

*He comes to an acceptance.* When a guy is first confronted by the need to supplement his T levels, he usually experiences an immediate knee-jerk reaction that meds are a bad thing to put into his body and that all meds are bad.

Over time, as a healthier, more confident version of himself emerges, his attitude changes. It's not that he wouldn't still prefer Door #1, but he comes to accept that Door #1 is closed and comes to peace with that. He looks at the remaining options of Door #2 or Door #3, and realizes that Door #3 is his best shot. T therapy simply becomes part of his life, like brushing his teeth and shaving.

*He puts a higher value on his marriage and his wife.* After a guy has been through the recovery process, he understands that marriage is fragile in a way he never did before and he realizes how much there is to lose. He has a new vision for what his marriage can be like and values the increased connection he's gained with his wife.

He also values his wife more. He sees the tremendous efforts she made on behalf of him and the marriage and the loyalty she exhibited in sticking with him through a tough time, and it makes him see her in a new light. You'll frequently hear a formerly low T guy talk about how grateful he is that his wife was willing to fight for him and not let the issue die.

***He respects himself more***. As he becomes a stronger, more confident leader, a man typically gains a new respect for himself that was missing during the low T years. He enjoys leading at work and at home. He engages with the kids in ways he didn't before and takes back the reins. As his wife, you are able to relax because you're no longer in this alone.

While he becomes more confident, in a strange way, he also becomes more humble. He realizes that he's not an island and that his actions, or failure to take action, impact his wife, his marriage, his family, his health, and his career.

What I hear over and over again is that he wishes he had found the solution earlier before so much damage had been done, that now that he's on the other side and things are so much better, he realizes how close to disaster things really were. He eventually comes to an acceptance that without the hard parts, he couldn't have achieved the gains he's made, and he comes to peace with that.

## You Have Changed

When you conquer difficult challenges in your life, it can't help but change you. When you first started down this path, you had no idea what was wrong in your marriage and no idea of whether it could get better. You took a leap of faith that you could make your marriage work and your work paid off. Your marriage is stronger and more passionate and vital than it's ever been. But while you hoped you could change your marriage, what you didn't count on was the way the journey would change *you*. That's a bonus. Like the prize in a box of Cracker Jacks. As you worked your way through the three steps in the *Recovery Stage*, a number of things happened:

***You've become stronger***. Overcoming obstacles makes you stronger and more resilient. You stop being a passive victim and learn to be clear about what you want and about what you are willing … and not willing … to accept. When you first started, you felt powerless and out of options. But you've learned that you do have options and you've learned that with enough energy, you do have the power to change your life.

You've also been tested. Some women in a low or no-sex marriage do not stay faithful. Let's be honest, it's tough to stay loyal when you feel like your husband doesn't care about you. But you had the perseverance to hang in there. That's a good thing to know about yourself.

***You got rid of your 'Good Girl'***. Somewhere along the way, you kicked her off the trail. You know … that good girl who wailed and complained but never took any action, the one who put everyone else's needs above her own and never set any boundaries, but then resented never getting any of her needs met. She's gone now and good riddance! May she rest in peace.

> **You've put a stake through the heart of your Good Girl.**

***You also lost the anger***. Once you take power back over your own life, you get rid of the anger. When you have the power to change your life, you don't have to be angry. You replace that sense of anger with a sense of achievement and strength. As a result, you no longer have rage bubbling just under the surface ready to leap forth at the earliest opportunity.

While most of the anger clears, there may still be some residual feelings of resentment that it took you so long to find the answers to the problems in your marriage. When I think of that girl I was sobbing by the side of the bathtub, I want to give her a swift kick in the pants and tell her to stop crying and get busy fixing her life! My guess is that when you look back at all the time you spent accepting a crappy marriage, you want to do the same.

You may find yourself having flashbacks in certain scenarios, and all those old feelings of rejection and anger come flooding back. I had one simple little mantra that helped, "It wasn't him, it wasn't me, it was just low T." Your husband wasn't trying to hurt you; he had a medical issue that affected his behavior. Now that the low T is fixed, he isn't the same person he was during those years when he rejected you so often, and you are not the same woman.

Unexpectedly, something else that helped was redecorating our bedroom. A seemingly insignificant act, but one with a big impact. Once the physical environment was different, we were more able to put the past behind us. You may find the same to be true for you. Throw on a new coat of paint, buy a new bedspread, rearrange your furniture, and see if it helps.

***You've become more attractive*** ... and I'm not talking simply about how you look. Increasing your energy and becoming happier is attractive. Instead of bubbling with anger, you now bubble with enthusiasm. People are attracted to positive energy. You're a lot more fun than you used to be and a lot more interesting.

***You've come to a place of acceptance.*** While you could mourn the 'wasted years', the truth is that those years weren't wasted. They were simply the cover charge you paid to become a stronger, more attractive version of you. You could not have achieved these gains without going through the struggles you faced in your marriage. You give up some short-term comfort to gain long-term advantages. That's a good thing.

## Your Lives Have Changed

As you go through the three-step process in the *Recovery Stage*, you find that your lives start changing. Low T is an energy vortex, it sucks energy out of both of you. The constant fights over the lack of sex multiply the effect. As you fix the medical and then move through each step of the recovery process, both of you gain energy. When you increase your energy, it has an impact on every facet of your life and you're able to move up to that next level.

**You will have more time**. One thing my husband and I found once we hit *Stage Five* is that we have a lot more time. All of those

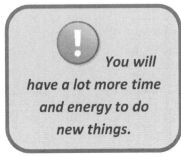

relationship discussions and late night arguments, in addition to being draining, take time. Now we use that time to better effect, planning our next home project, discussing issues about the kids, talking about career development, or simply dreaming about what we want our future to look like. It's so much a better use of our time!

**You will feel ready for the next challenge**. One surprising thing we both noticed is that once we left the angst of the low T recovery behind, we were a bit ... *restless*. All of that drama, even though it was negative, was stimulating! We didn't really want to settle into a nice, boring rut ... so we didn't. Instead, we both found that we were ready for the next level. We invested a lot of our newfound energy into our careers with good results. We started planning for a new house. My husband started a new martial art and I stepped up my workouts in a new gym. All those things that had been put on hold during the dark years gained a new priority. It was our own personal Renaissance.

## No Going Back

It takes much more energy to put an object into motion than to keep it moving. It's the same with a low T marriage. Getting through the three steps of the *Recovery Stage* does take a tremendous amount of energy. Keeping it locked in is much easier; however, it does still take *some* effort. You can't go back to the low energy state you started in.

At first, you will find yourself bouncing in and out of *Stage Five*. Don't feel defeated by that. While you will bounce for a while before eventually stabilizing, you will never go back to those dark low T days. Keep tracking your marital satisfaction and over time, you'll realize that your marriage momentum is gradually increasing even though there are peaks and valleys throughout the process.

Keep doing the energy and attraction-boosting activities in *Step Two* and the marriage-building tools in *Step Three*. There will be times, of course, when life gets busy, but if you incorporate these activities into your daily life so that they are part of your routine, you will find it much easier to keep your marriage momentum going.

# A Gift Beyond Measure

Some people believe that things happen for a reason. I don't know whether that's true; *sometimes bad things just happen*, like cancer and polio. I do know, however, that each of us will face challenges in this life one way or another, whether it's low T or infidelity or addiction or cancer. And those challenges will test who we are. You can complain bitterly and do nothing, or you can rise to the challenge and change your outcome to the best of your ability.

The challenges we encounter also shape who we are. I am a different person than I was six years ago. I am less passive and more direct, and I have a firmer grasp on what I want out of life.

The challenges of the low T years have made me incredibly grateful for my good health and I recognize it for the blessing it is. I get up every day thankful that my body is strong and active and will do what I want it to do.

I am so glad to have the knowledge to help my four boys stay healthy and maintain a lifestyle that keeps their testosterone levels optimal. Hopefully, they and their future wives will never go through what my husband and I did.

I am also hugely grateful that I have a chance to help people who are struggling as I was a few years ago. I am passionate about working with people who want to live a healthy lifestyle, and it is immensely satisfying to help people avoid the mistakes my husband and I made and watch them rebuild their lives and marriages.

I believe that low testosterone is a neglected medical issue and needs more research. When you think about how many health conditions are associated with low testosterone, it seems unbelievable that it hasn't been studied in more depth. I think that will all change as our population ages, and I am grateful to be able to speak from my experience and spread the word to help other people.

So as you can see, in a strange way, low T was a gift, although I didn't recognize it as such at the time. It has taken me places I otherwise never would have gone and it's made all the difference in my life. My hope is that I've helped you get to a place where you can look back and say the same.

# What to Expect at this Point

- *You will cycle in and out of Stage Five for a while. These cycles will come less and less frequently as you gain stability.*
- *Arguments, when they happen, tend to be more productive and less bitter.*
- *His T levels are nice and stable and he feels great!*
- *He has taken over the reins of keeping track of and ordering his own labs and meds.*
- *He is taking more of a leadership role with the family.*
- *Both of you have become more productive; you can't believe how much you are getting done at work and at home.*
- *You feel more connected and bonded to him and you enjoy being with him.*
- *You may even fall in love with your husband all over again.*
- *He initiates much more frequently; there are actually (gasp!) times when he wants sex more than you do. This makes you really happy. Sex is more intense and passionate.*

# Action Steps

- *Recognize and accept that both of you have been changed by your experiences with low T.*

- *Accept that you will still sometimes have flashes of anger and he will sometimes have feelings of regret over the years that you 'lost' to low T. Remind yourself that for everything you gave up, you got so much more in return.*
- *Keep tracking your marital satisfaction as an early warning detection system. If satisfaction decreases substantially, go back and look for the blockages.*
- *Keep using the tools from Steps One, Two and Three to keep momentum growing.*
- *Enjoy your high T marriage!*

# Glossary

**Albumin** - a protein that binds to testosterone, although not as strongly as SHBG

**Bioavailable testosterone -** the combination of free testosterone plus the amount of testosterone weakly bound to albumin that can easily break free

**Clomid** - an estrogen receptor agonist/antagonist that increases testosterone production by blocking estrogen receptors and preventing estrogen conversion

**Compounding pharmacy** - a pharmacy where the pharmacist makes your medication 'from scratch', mixing individual ingredients together based on what your doctor has prescribed

**Continuous positive airway pressure machine** (CPAP) – a small machine that has a mask that fits over the nose and/or mouth and provides continuous pressure in order to keep the airway open while sleeping

**DHEA** (Dehydroepiandrosterone) - a hormone produced in the adrenal glands and a precursor to testosterone

**DHT (dihydrotestosterone)** - a strong male hormone produced by the conversion of testosterone

**Edging** - deliberately engaging in sexual stimulation without finishing to orgasm in order to increase sexual desire

**Endogenous testosterone** - testosterone made internally by a man's own body

**Erythocytosis -** increase in red blood cells

**Ester** – carbon molecule added to testosterone to slow the release of the testosterone from the injection site into the blood stream

**Estrogen** - a hormone made in men and women's bodies that is key to bone health and sexual function, amongst other things

**Exogenous testosterone** – testosterone added from an external source

**Follicle stimulating hormone (FSH)** – a hormone produced by the pituitary gland that stimulates the testes to produce sperm

**Free testosterone** - the amount of unbound testosterone  actually available to be used by the body

**Free T3 and T4** - additional thyroid measures that give a picture of how the thyroid is performing

**Gonadotropin-releasing hormone (GnRH)** - a hormone produced by the hypothalamus gland that stimulates the pituitary gland to produce luteinizing hormone (LH) and follicle-stimulating hormone (FSH)

**Gynecomastia** - enlargement of a man's breasts, often caused by elevated estrogen

**Hormone** - a chemical produced in your body that is transported to different areas  via the bloodstream, where it produces different types of responses

**Human chorionic gonadotropin** (HCG) – a hormone produced by the human body that closely mimics luteinizing hormone and stimulates natural testosterone production

**Hypogonadism, combination**- low testosterone whose cause originates in both the testes and the hypothalamus-pituitary axis

**Hypogonadism, primary** - low testosterone whose cause originates in the testes

**Hypogonadism, secondary** - low testosterone whose cause originates in the hypothalamus-pituitary axis

**Hypothalamus-Pituitary-Gonadal (HPG) axis** – Glands that work together to produce testosterone and sperm

**Hypothalamus gland** - a gland in the brain responsible for releasing GnRH to signal the pituitary to produce LH and FSH

**Hypothyroid** - low thyroid function

**Intramuscular** (IM) – an injection administered shallowly into muscle tissue

**Leydig cells** – cells in the testes that produce testosterone

**Libido -** sex drive

**Luteinizing hormone (LH)** - a hormone produced by the pituitary gland that stimulates the Leydig cells in the testes to produce testosterone

**Neuroplasticity** - changes in the neural pathways in the brain due to changes in behavior, environment, thinking, emotions, hormones, and nutrition

**Off-label medicine** - a medicine used to treat people with a condition other than the one for which the medicine was approved

**PDE-5 inhibitors** - a drug used to produce or enhance erections

**PIV** - penis in vagina, another term for sexual intercourse

**Polycythemia** – increase in red cell mass

**Premature ejaculation (PE)** - inability to delay ejaculation during intercourse

**Priapism** - an erection that won't subside

**PSA** (Prostate Specific Antigen) – measures a protein produced by the prostate gland. Elevated levels can indicate prostate problems and be a contraindication for testosterone therapy.

**Refractory period** (recovery phase) - a time period immediately after sex during which a man becomes uninterested in and possibly incapable of having sex again

**Sex hormone binding globulin (SHBG)** - a protein that binds testosterone and renders it unusable

**Sexual dysfunction, erectile dysfunction, impotence** - often used interchangeably to refer to a man's inability to get or keep an erection long enough for satisfactory sex

**Sleep apnea** - a condition characterized by shallow breathing or pauses in breathing while sleeping; sleep apnea often contributes to low testosterone

**Sub Q** (subcutaneously) – an injection administered just under the skin

**Testes (gonads)** - twin glands that produce testosterone and sperm

**Testosterone** - a steroid hormone produced mainly in a man's testicles, with much smaller amounts produced by the adrenal glands

**Thyroid stimulating hormone** (TSH) - a measure of thyroid function; thyroid problems tend to go hand in hand with testosterone problems

**Total Testosterone** - a measure of testosterone that includes all testosterone, whether bound or unbound by proteins

**Transdermal** - a medicine which is absorbed through the skin

# Recommended Resources

## Books on Low Testosterone and T therapy

**Morgentaler, Abraham, MD.** *Testosterone for Life: Recharge Your Vitality, Sex Drive, Muscle Mass & Overall Health!* New York: McGraw-Hill, 2009. Print.

Excellent overview of testosterone and T therapy with an excellent chapter on the relationship between testosterone and prostate cancer and why the medical establishment got it wrong for so long

**Shippen, Eugene, MD and William Fryer.** *The Testosterone Syndrome:  The Critical Factor For Energy, Health, & Sexuality – Reversing The Male Menopause.* Lanham: M. Evans, 2007. Print.

Another good overview of testosterone production, plus a must-read chapter on the connection between testosterone and cardiovascular health

**Teeple, Sloan, MD and Susan Teeple.** *I'm Still Sexy So What's Up with Him?* New York: Morgan James, 2012. Print.

Written by a doctor who was himself diagnosed with low testosterone after being urged by his wife to find out what was going on with him. Adds a very nice human element along with the more usual medical viewpoint.

**Vergel, Nelson, BsChE, MBA.** *What You Need To Know About Your Man's Testosterone.* Houston: Milestones, 2011. Print.

Nelson Vergel struggled with low T himself, and is a passionate advocate for safely using testosterone therapy. A good overview of low testosterone with helpful detail on how to actually administer T therapy, plus an excellent chapter on treating erectile dysfunction

# High T Marriage

**Glover, Robert, PhD.** *No More Mr. Nice Guy.* Philadelphia: Running Press, 2000. Print.

A good guide on teaching men to set boundaries.

**Kay, Athol.** *The Mindful Attraction Plan: Your Practical Roadmap to Creating the Life, Love and Success You Want.* CreateSpace, 2013. Print.

A great resource on improving the energy in your life and marriage. Geared to both men and women, it gives excellent insight on how to take the steps that will change your life.

**Kay, Athol.** *The Married Guy's Guide to Wife.* Internet video.

After a long-term period of low testosterone, a man often has a tough time regaining his confidence and his ability to attract his wife. This is an excellent video series on attracting your wife and becoming the strong leader she wants to follow.

Currently a video series and soon available in book form.

# Neuroplasticity

**Leaf, Caroline, PhD.** *Who Switched Off My Brain? Controlling Toxic Thoughts and Emotions*. Dallas: Switch on Your Brain, 2007. Print.

# Sexual Technique

**Kerner, Ian, PhD.** *She Comes First: The Thinking Man's Guide to Pleasuring a Woman*. New York: ReganBooks, 2004. Print.

**Silverberg, Sy, MD.** *Lasting Longer: The Treatment Program for Premature Ejaculation*. 2nd ed. Canada: SWS, 2010. Print.

# About the Author

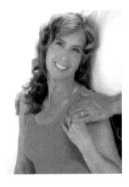

I specialize in helping people who are struggling with low testosterone. This includes guys who have just found out that their T levels are low and are looking for lifestyle changes that will help turn it back around, women who are trying to figure out why their husbands have lost interest in sex, and couples who are working to overcome low T and get their marriage back on track.

Having beat low testosterone in my own marriage, one of my favorite things to do is to help other people do the same. I get a lot of satisfaction from helping people save time and money by avoiding the pitfalls and detours my husband and I experienced in our own low T journey.

Low testosterone takes a tremendous toll on a couple, and marriages don't always survive it. My mission is to help your marriage not only survive low T, but also thrive!

I live with my husband and five kids outside Atlanta, where I wade through the bedlam every day, trying to keep my chocolate stash from the ravening hordes. I am not always successful at this as I am sadly out-numbered.

In the midst of all the mayhem, my husband and I frequently take time to shut our bedroom door on the chaos and enjoy our high T marriage!

# About Coaching

## When You Need Help Putting it All Together

If you are struggling in a low T marriage and need help moving forward, I'll be glad to coach you through it. I coach a variety of people ... from wives who can't get their husbands to check their T levels ... to men who are simply tired of living a half-life and want to feel good again ... to couples who are having a tough time getting past the hurt and anger of the dark years of low T.

Sometimes a woman just needs me to tell her that she's not crazy for wanting a healthy sex life with her husband. Sometimes she needs to hear that she's not alone and that it's not hopeless, that other people have been through what she's going through and made it to the other side.

I also coach men who want help figuring out what their levels mean and what their next step is. They also need reassurance that this isn't the end of the world, that guys can beat low T and regain their energy and vitality.

Couples also need help with the medical process, but in addition, they frequently contact me because they're ready to move on to the *Recovery Stage* and get their marriage back on track.

Whatever your reasons for wanting coaching, know that I am a safe, confidential, listening ear who can help you make a plan for moving forward and getting out of the low T mire.

You can contact me with questions via e-mail or my blog. Drop me a line, I'd love to hear your story.

rebeccawatson.serenity@gmail.com
www.highTmarriage.com

Printed in Great Britain
by Amazon

60184610R00175